The Antidepressant Taper Handbook

A Plain-English Guide to Coming Off SSRIs, SNRIs, Mirtazapine, and Trazodone Safely

With Withdrawal Symptom Maps, Hyperbolic Tapering Schedules, and Conversation Scripts for Your Prescriber

Charles Tadelesh Prada

This book is intended solely for general educational and informational purposes. It is not a substitute for professional medical advice, diagnosis, or treatment. Nothing in this book should be construed as instruction to start, stop, reduce, or change the dose of any prescribed medication without the direct supervision of a qualified prescriber. Antidepressant tapering carries real risks and must be undertaken in partnership with a healthcare professional who knows your history and can respond to changes in your condition. Always consult your prescribing clinician before beginning, adjusting, or ending any pharmacological treatment, and continue to work with them throughout the process.

All patient descriptions in this book are composite illustrations created for educational purposes. Names, biographical details, dosing histories, and clinical situations have been changed or invented to protect confidentiality. Any resemblance to a specific individual is coincidental.

The author and publisher make no representations or warranties with respect to the accuracy, applicability, or completeness of the content. Individual responses to antidepressant withdrawal vary enormously and no book can predict how any particular person's nervous system will respond to a taper. The author and publisher disclaim any liability for loss or risk incurred as a consequence, directly or indirectly, of the use or application of any of the material in this book. Readers assume full responsibility for their own decisions regarding their medical care.

If you are experiencing thoughts of self-harm or suicide, please reach out immediately. In the United States, call or text 988 for the Suicide and Crisis Lifeline. In the United Kingdom and Republic of Ireland, call Samaritans on 116 123. In other countries, please contact your local emergency service or crisis line. You do not have to face this alone, and help is available at any hour.

First edition. Published 2026.

ISBN: 979-8-90599-193-6

Staten House

Table of Contents

Preface

I did not train as a taper specialist. Almost nobody did. What I trained for was ordinary mental health care, the kind that happens in clinics and consulting rooms, and for years I did what most of us were taught to do. I helped people start antidepressants when they seemed to need them. I checked in about side effects. I renewed prescriptions. And when someone said, after a year or three or ten, that they wanted to try coming off, I told them what the guidelines told me to tell them. Halve the dose for two weeks. Then stop. If anything feels off, come back and we will restart.

For a long time, I did not question this. And then I met the people for whom two weeks was catastrophically insufficient.

They came back after their attempted taper looking hollowed out. Some described sensations they could not name, brief electric-shock feelings in the head, floors that seemed to tilt, a nausea that would not settle. Some told me that a rage they had never felt before was living in their chest. Some had not slept properly for a month. And when I did what I had been taught to do, when I told them that this was probably their original condition returning and that we should restart the medication, some of them looked at me with an expression I still remember. It was the expression of a person who has been told that what they are experiencing is not real.

This handbook is the book I wish I had been able to give them.

It is a book about what is known now, in 2026, about how to come off certain antidepressants without collapsing your nervous system, and about how to tell the difference between withdrawal and the return of the condition the drug was treating. It is not an anti-medication book. Some of my patients need their antidepressant, and some will need it for the rest of their lives, and there is no shame in that. It is not a wellness book either. It will not tell you that the answer is turmeric or gratitude journals or cold plunges. It is a practical handbook for a specific decision: you want to come off, or you want to try, and you need a plan that respects both the pharmacology and the fact that you have a life to keep running while you do it.

The plan in this book rests on a body of work that has grown up over the past decade. The clinicians and researchers who did the hardest part of that work include Mark Horowitz, David Taylor, Anders Sørensen, Giovanni Fava, Michael Hengartner, and Adele Framer, along with the many thousands of patients whose forum posts on Surviving Antidepressants first mapped what the literature was slow to see. My debt to them is significant, and their sources are listed at the back. Nothing in this book is my personal opinion where a better source exists.

A word about tone. If you are reading this, you have almost certainly been dismissed by someone. Perhaps a doctor, perhaps a family member, perhaps a version of yourself that decided a while ago that being sensitive to a small pill was ridiculous. I am not going to dismiss you. I am also not going to catastrophise on your behalf. Coming off an antidepressant is a real thing that real people do successfully every day, at a pace their nervous system can follow. Let us work out what that pace looks like for you.

How to Use This Book

Before you start reading in earnest, a few practical notes about how the book is put together and how to get the most out of it.

The book is organised into three broad sections. Chapters 1 through 6 give you the shared foundations: what the drugs are, what the four key words mean, why standard tapers fail, whether now is the right time for you, how to draft a plan, and how to solve the formulation problem. Chapters 7 through 9 give you drug-specific schedules and details for each of the ten medications the book covers. Chapters 10 through 16 walk you through the actual experience of the taper: what symptoms to expect, how to tell withdrawal from relapse, how to make the hold-slow-reinstate decision, what to do if the syndrome becomes protracted, how to talk to your prescriber, how to keep the rest of your life running, and what the first year off tends to look like. The appendices are practical reference tools: worksheets, decision aids, glossary, resources, and further reading.

If you are just starting to think about tapering, read the book front to back. The chapters build on each other, and each one assumes you have absorbed the ones before it.

If you are already partway into a taper and something has gone wrong, the fastest path to a useful answer is often to jump to Chapter 11 (withdrawal or relapse), Chapter 12 (hold, slow, or reinstate), or Chapter 10 (the symptom map), depending on what your specific question is. Come back to the earlier chapters later, once the immediate situation is stable.

If you are supporting someone else through their taper, Appendix J is written for you specifically. The rest of the book is still useful, but Appendix J is where you will find the most direct guidance.

If you are a prescriber or nurse using this book as a reference for a patient, the chapters that will most repay your time are Chapter 3 (the pharmacological case for hyperbolic tapering), the drug-specific chapter for your patient's medication, and Appendix E (the one-page evidence summary designed for prescriber use).

The worksheets in Appendix A and the symptom log in Appendix B are meant to be copied and used. If you have this book in physical form, copy them into a notebook or spreadsheet. If you have it in digital form, transcribe them into whatever tool you prefer. The value is in the daily use, not in the format.

A note on the schedules in Chapters 7, 8, and 9. Every schedule in this book is an example. It is not a prescription and it is not a rigid rule. The purpose of each schedule is to give you a concrete starting point that reflects the pharmacology of your specific drug. Every real taper will diverge from the schedule at some point, and that is normal. What matters is the underlying pattern (hyperbolic reductions that get smaller as the dose gets smaller, intervals that give your nervous system time to settle), not the specific milligram values on any given line.

A note on the case examples throughout the book. The patients described in these examples are composites, drawn from clinical experience and modified to protect confidentiality. Names, biographical details, dosing histories, and specific clinical situations have been changed or invented. Any resemblance to a specific individual is coincidental. What is not invented is the underlying pattern of what happens during tapers, which is drawn from patterns that recur across many patients and across the clinical literature.

A note on language. This book is written in British English, with occasional accommodation for American English where terminology differs. Where a drug has different brand names in different countries, both are given. Where clinical practices vary internationally, I have tried to note the variation.

A final note. The book is deliberately not written in the register of medical advice. It is written in the register of a thoughtful clinician talking to a thoughtful reader, at the pace and depth of a real conversation. If you find yourself wanting to argue with something in it, that is a good sign; you should argue with it, out loud or silently, and see whether your objection changes your plan. Nothing in this book is meant to override your own judgement, or your prescriber's judgement, about what is right for you. It is meant to give you the raw material for both of your judgements to work with.

Now, to the introduction.

Why This Book

There is a specific conversation that happens in family doctor surgeries and psychiatric offices all over the English-speaking world, and it goes something like this. A patient has been on a common antidepressant for anywhere between six months and twenty years. The reason they started may have been depression, or generalised anxiety, or panic, or postpartum mood changes, or grief, or some combination of the above. Life is now more stable, or less exhausting, or in some other way different from what it was, and the patient wants to try coming off. They raise this with their prescriber. The prescriber, who is often kind and well-intentioned and working under time pressure, produces a taper plan.

The plan is almost always some version of the same thing. Halve the dose for two to four weeks. Then stop. If anything happens, we will restart.

For some patients, that plan works. Withdrawal, if it occurs, is mild and short-lived. Life goes on.

For a large minority of patients, the plan does not work at all. What happens instead is a cascade of physical, sensory, sleep, and emotional symptoms that begins somewhere between the second day and the second month after the dose reduction. These symptoms are often written off, by the patient themselves or by the prescriber, as the original condition returning. The patient is put back on the drug, sometimes at a higher dose than before, and stays on it for another year, or another decade, or forever. The word failure does not quite capture what has happened, because failure implies that the plan was ever workable in the first place. What has actually happened is that a plan drawn up in an era before we understood the pharmacology of these drugs at low doses has failed to meet a patient whose nervous system does not run on the timetable the leaflet describes.

That is the situation this book is trying to address.

Who this book is for

This book is for adults currently on a selective serotonin reuptake inhibitor, a serotonin and norepinephrine reuptake inhibitor, mirtazapine, or trazodone who want to try coming off, or who have tried and hit something they did not expect. It is also for the family member or partner who is trying to help. It is also, quietly, for the prescriber or nurse who wants to hand a patient something the patient can read at home and come back to the next appointment prepared.

It covers, in depth:

sertraline, escitalopram, citalopram, fluoxetine, paroxetine, venlafaxine, duloxetine, desvenlafaxine, mirtazapine, and trazodone.

It does not cover, in this edition:

tricyclic antidepressants, monoamine oxidase inhibitors, bupropion, ketamine, esketamine, benzodiazepines, z-drugs, antipsychotics, mood stabilisers, or stimulants. Some of the principles will still apply to those medications, but the drug-specific chapters will not be useful to you if you are on one of them. Find a book, a clinician, or a peer community that specialises in the drug you are actually on.

Who this book is not for

This book is not for anyone considering stopping an antidepressant without the involvement of a prescriber. There are two reasons for this. The first is safety. Withdrawal can produce agitation, sleep collapse, and in some people an increase in suicidal thoughts, and you should not face that without medical support. The second is that many of the tools in this book, particularly the small-dose formulations and the reinstatement options, are only accessible through a prescriber. Working without one leaves you without your main lever.

If your current prescriber is not willing to support a slow taper, that is a solvable problem, and Chapter 14 will help you work on it. What you should not do is proceed alone.

How to read this book

The book is arranged so that reading it front to back gives you a full understanding of what you are doing and why. If you are the kind of reader who likes to know the map before you take the first step, do that.

If you are impatient, or if you are already partway into a taper and need a specific answer today, here is the shortcut. Read Chapter 3, which explains why standard tapers fail and what hyperbolic tapering is, then read whichever of Chapters 7, 8, or 9 covers your specific drug. That will give you the minimum information you need to draft a plan and take it to your prescriber. Then, after your appointment, come back and read the rest. You will need Chapter 10, on withdrawal symptoms, and Chapter 12, on when to hold, slow, or reinstate, before you get very far into the taper itself.

A note about certainty

Some of what is in this book is well established. The receptor occupancy science, the drug half-lives, the general principle that longer users need slower tapers, the fact that withdrawal exists at all: these things are no longer seriously contested in the research literature.

Some of what is in this book is less well established. The precise best step-down for any given drug is still an area of active study. The base rate of protracted withdrawal is estimated from patient reports rather than from randomised trials, and estimates vary considerably. The optimal length of a hold when symptoms emerge is a matter of clinical judgement more than fixed protocol. Where I am summarising something that is contested, I will tell you so. Where I am giving you a number, I will tell you where the number came from.

You do not need certainty to plan a taper. You need to know what is likely, what is possible, and what to do when the picture changes.

A note about safety

Antidepressant withdrawal, and the taper process itself, can be associated with an increase in mood volatility, agitation, and, for some people, thoughts of self-harm. This is a documented phenomenon and it is not a sign that you are weak, broken, or beyond help. It is a signal that your nervous system is under stress and that you need more support, not less.

If, at any point during the process this book describes, you find yourself having thoughts of ending your life, please stop and reach out. Call your prescriber. Call your emergency crisis line. In the United States, call or text 988. In the United Kingdom and Ireland, call Samaritans on 116 123, or call NHS 111. In other countries, use your local equivalent. If someone is with you, tell them what is happening. You do not need to be certain that you are in crisis in order to reach for help. Reaching for help early is what keeps a difficult few weeks from becoming something worse.

What you will have when you finish

By the last page, you will have:

a clear mental model of what your drug is doing and why coming off it is not the same as never having started; a written taper plan drawn up around the pharmacology of your specific drug; a formulation strategy that lets you actually reduce by the amounts the plan calls for; a symptom log you have been keeping across the taper; a set of decision rules for the moments when things do not go according to plan; a small library of scripts for the conversations you will need to have with your prescriber; and a realistic picture of what life on the other side of the last dose tends to look like.

You will not have certainty. Nobody has certainty about this. What you will have is a way of proceeding that respects both the science and the fact that you are a person with a life to live.

Turn the page.

Chapter 1: What You Are Actually On

Bindi had been on citalopram for nine years when she came in to talk about coming off. She was 41. She had started the drug during her first pregnancy, when a persistent low mood and morning tearfulness had frightened her enough to ask for help, and she had never quite got round to stopping. Her son was eight now. Her marriage was steady. Work was fine. When she sat down in the chair opposite me and said, "I think I'd like to try being me again," I understood exactly what she meant.

I asked her what she knew about the drug she had been taking every day for nearly a decade. She thought for a moment. "It's an SSRI," she said. "It stops my brain from getting rid of the serotonin. I know it takes a while to build up when you start. I don't know if it takes a while to leave."

That was more than most patients could tell me. It was still not enough to plan a taper on.

Before you plan how to come off a medication, you need a working understanding of what the medication is doing, what family it belongs to, and how quickly your body clears it. You do not need a pharmacology degree. You need enough to make sense of what happens next.

The four families this book covers

The antidepressants covered by this book fall into four functional groups.

The largest group is the selective serotonin reuptake inhibitors, always shortened to SSRIs. This group includes sertraline, escitalopram, citalopram, fluoxetine, and paroxetine, along with a few less commonly prescribed cousins. What all SSRIs share is that they slow down the reuptake of serotonin at the synapse, meaning that serotonin sits in the gap between nerve cells for longer and has more chance to signal. Over time, the brain adapts to this by adjusting the number and sensitivity of its serotonin receptors. When the drug is removed, the brain has to unlearn those adaptations, and until it does, the machinery is out of tune. That out-of-tuneness is what we call withdrawal.

The second group is the serotonin and norepinephrine reuptake inhibitors, always shortened to SNRIs. This group includes venlafaxine (Effexor), duloxetine (Cymbalta), and desvenlafaxine (Pristiq). SNRIs do to norepinephrine what SSRIs do to serotonin, and they do it at the same time as they act on serotonin. This dual action can be helpful for certain conditions, but it also means that when the drug is removed, two neurotransmitter systems need to re-adjust rather than one. In practice, this often makes SNRI withdrawal feel more intense than SSRI withdrawal, and it makes venlafaxine in particular one of the hardest antidepressants in common use to stop taking.

The third and fourth groups sit slightly apart. Mirtazapine acts primarily on a set of receptors called alpha-2 adrenergic receptors, along with certain histamine and serotonin receptors, in ways that increase norepinephrine and serotonin release. It is often prescribed for depression combined with poor sleep because its histamine-blocking effect at low doses is strongly sedating. Trazodone is technically classified as a serotonin antagonist and reuptake inhibitor, but in practice it is prescribed most often at low doses for sleep, because it too has strong sedating effects at low doses. Both drugs behave differently in the body from the SSRIs and SNRIs, and both produce their own characteristic patterns when tapered, especially around sleep.

You do not need to memorise this. You need to know which of the four groups your drug belongs to, because the taper plans in Chapters 7, 8, and 9 are organised around those groups.

Half-life, and why it matters more than you think

Half-life is the length of time it takes your body to reduce the concentration of a drug by half after you stop taking it. It is measured in hours. Most people never encounter the concept in ordinary life, but if you are planning a taper, half-life is the single most useful number in your drug's pharmacology.

The rule of thumb is straightforward. Drugs with short half-lives leave the body quickly, which means their concentration in the blood swings widely between doses, which means that even a small dose reduction can produce a large and rapid drop in effect at the receptor. Drugs with long half-lives leave the body slowly, which means their concentration is steadier between doses, which means dose reductions are cushioned in time.

Compare venlafaxine and fluoxetine. Venlafaxine has a half-life of around five hours. Fluoxetine has an active metabolite with a half-life of one to two weeks. In practical terms, if you take your venlafaxine at 8am on Monday and forget your Tuesday dose, by Tuesday evening the drug in your system has already dropped substantially, and by Wednesday morning you may be in acute withdrawal. If you do the same thing with fluoxetine, you will very likely not notice for days. Fluoxetine is not a gentler drug because someone made it that way. Its half-life is doing the work.

This has three implications you should keep in mind as you read the rest of the book. First, missed doses of short-half-life drugs are not neutral events; they are small, unplanned tapers in miniature. Second, drugs with short half-lives generally need slower, more careful tapering schedules than drugs with long half-lives. Third, this is the reason a fluoxetine bridge is sometimes considered when tapering off a difficult short-half-life drug like paroxetine or venlafaxine, a technique we will come back to in Chapter 6.

> **Important Point:** *Short half-life is the single strongest predictor of a difficult taper. If your drug has a half-life of less than twelve hours, plan to go slower than the leaflet suggests.*

Which drugs tend to be hard, which tend to be gentler

Withdrawal severity varies from person to person and cannot be predicted with certainty. That said, the accumulated clinical and patient experience of the past two decades has produced a reasonably consistent ranking.

Paroxetine (Paxil, Seroxat) has the reputation of being the hardest SSRI to stop. Its half-life is short by SSRI standards, at around 21 hours, and it has active affinity for the muscarinic receptor system as well, which adds a set of anticholinergic withdrawal symptoms that other SSRIs do not produce. Many patients who tapered paroxetine successfully describe schedules that lasted a year or more.

Venlafaxine (Effexor) has the reputation of being the hardest antidepressant in common use to stop, full stop. Its half-life is around five hours, its parent compound and its active metabolite have somewhat different pharmacology, and the discontinuation symptoms are frequently intense and rapid in onset. Patients who miss a single dose often notice withdrawal within hours. Duloxetine (Cymbalta) sits close behind venlafaxine, for similar reasons.

Sertraline (Zoloft), citalopram (Celexa), and escitalopram (Cipralex, Lexapro) sit in the middle of the range. Withdrawal is common on rapid tapers but is generally more manageable than paroxetine or venlafaxine on well-planned slow tapers. Their half-lives are longer, in the range of 25 to 35 hours, which cushions dose changes somewhat.

Fluoxetine (Prozac) is the gentlest of the SSRIs to stop, largely because of its long half-life. Many patients can taper fluoxetine over shorter timeframes than the other SSRIs without significant symptoms. This is also why fluoxetine is used, in some circumstances, as a bridge drug during a taper off a harder-to-stop antidepressant.

Mirtazapine and trazodone are their own case. The withdrawal syndrome from these two drugs is dominated by sleep disturbance, because both drugs are strongly sedating at the low doses at which they are commonly used. Coming off them without a sleep-collapse plan is the single most common reason attempts fail. We will spend a full chapter on this in Chapter 9.

None of this means your particular experience will follow the ranking. Some patients taper paroxetine smoothly. Some patients hit unexpected walls on sertraline. The ranking is useful for planning, not for predicting.

The drug's therapeutic effect and its withdrawal effect are not the same thing

One of the most damaging assumptions in the older thinking about antidepressant withdrawal is that if a symptom emerges when the drug is reduced, and that symptom looks anything like the condition the drug was originally treating, then the drug must still be needed. In other words, if you started an SSRI for anxiety, and you have anxiety when you cut the dose, then you have "relapsed" and should go back on the drug.

This reasoning is neat, and it is often wrong. The condition that responds to a drug and the withdrawal syndrome that emerges when the drug is stopped are two different biological events, and they can produce overlapping symptoms without being the same thing.

We will return to this distinction in Chapter 11, which is entirely devoted to telling withdrawal apart from relapse. For now, hold the idea loosely. The fact that you feel anxious a week after a dose reduction does not automatically mean your anxiety is back. It may mean that; it may mean that your brain is temporarily under-serotonergic while it re-adapts; it may mean both are happening at once. The point is that the meaning of the symptom is not obvious from the symptom alone.

What this book does not cover

A quick note on scope, so you are not surprised later.

This book does not cover tricyclic antidepressants such as amitriptyline, nortriptyline, clomipramine, and imipramine, and it does not cover monoamine oxidase inhibitors such as phenelzine or moclobemide. These are older classes of drug with distinct withdrawal profiles and, in the case of MAOIs, significant safety considerations around switching. If you are on one of these, you need a source that specialises in them.

It also does not cover bupropion (Wellbutrin, Zyban) in depth. Bupropion works on norepinephrine and dopamine rather than serotonin, and its withdrawal syndrome is milder and shorter for most people than the drugs in this book. A brief note appears in the introduction to Chapter 7, but it will not give you a full taper plan.

It does not cover benzodiazepines, z-drugs, antipsychotics, mood stabilisers, or stimulants, all of which are sometimes prescribed alongside antidepressants but each of which has its own separate pharmacology and its own separate literature.

Your personal drug profile

Before you go further, take a moment to write down the following, either in the margin of this book, in a notebook, or on a page in the app of your choice. You are going to need this information for every subsequent chapter.

The drug you are on, by generic name and by brand name if you know it. The dose you are currently taking. The formulation, meaning tablet, capsule, or liquid, and whether it is standard release or extended release. The length of time you have been on it, to the nearest year. Any past attempts to come off, what happened, and how long each attempt lasted. Your reason for wanting to come off now.

This is the raw material of your plan. Bindi's version, when we put it together, was: citalopram, 20 mg, tablet, nine years, no prior attempts, wanting to feel her own emotional range again. It is not a fancy piece of paper. It is enough to work with.

Bindi's next step

I told Bindi we were not going to design her taper that first appointment. We were going to spend two more sessions understanding what she was on, why it had helped, whether it was still helping, and what a realistic taper timeline would look like. I told her the honest headline: a citalopram taper from 20 mg with nine years of use behind it was likely to take a year or longer if we did it in a way her nervous system could follow. She thought about this and then said, "That is more than I expected. But it is also less than I feared." I told her this was the correct response, and that the fear the taper would take five years, or that it would break her, was not supported by anything we knew, but that neither was the assumption that four weeks would do it.

She agreed to come back the following week having read the equivalent of Chapters 1 and 2 of this book, and having drafted her personal drug profile. That was the beginning of her taper, not the beginning of her dose reductions. There is a difference, and it matters.

The Key Point of this chapter, which I ask you to carry with you into the next: you are not tapering a general category called antidepressants. You are tapering a specific molecule with a specific half-life and a specific withdrawal profile, and the plan you draw up needs to reflect that.

If you skip this step, you will draw up a plan that is generic. Generic plans fail. Specific plans, patiently followed, tend not to.

In the next chapter, we will look at the terms that are used to describe what happens when antidepressants are stopped, because if you cannot name what is happening, you cannot talk about it clearly with anyone, and the conversation with your prescriber is a large part of what makes the difference.

Chapter 2: Four Words Kept Straight

The most consequential conversation of a taper is often not the one where you draw up the schedule. It is the one where you and your prescriber try to describe what is happening when you feel unwell after a dose reduction. If you use the wrong word, the entire treatment plan changes. If your prescriber uses the wrong word, so does your medical record.

Four words tend to get shuffled together, and shuffling them together is the source of a great deal of avoidable suffering. The words are dependence, addiction, withdrawal, and relapse. Each one describes a different thing. Each one carries a different clinical implication. Getting them straight will help you advocate for yourself, understand what your prescriber means when they speak, and know what you are asking for when you ask for it.

Physical dependence

Physical dependence is the state that develops when a body has become physiologically adapted to the ongoing presence of a substance and would react in some way if that substance were suddenly removed. This is not a moral or psychological condition. It is a biological one, and it can develop with a wide range of legitimate medications. People are physically dependent on their blood pressure medication in the sense that stopping it would cause their blood pressure to rise. People are physically dependent on their thyroid replacement in the sense that stopping it would cause their thyroid hormone levels to drop. Neither situation is called addiction, and neither situation carries the stigma of addiction, because in both cases the dependence is understood to be an expected biological adaptation to a substance the body needs.

Antidepressants produce physical dependence in a substantial proportion of people who take them for more than a few months. This is now the mainstream view in the medical literature, and it is one of the most important pieces of language shift of the past decade. The current view is that the withdrawal symptoms people describe when they reduce or stop an antidepressant are the direct consequence of a nervous system that has adapted to the presence of the drug and is now having to unadapt.

Recognising physical dependence does not tell you anything about whether the drug should have been prescribed, whether it is still helping, or whether the person should be trying to come off. It only tells you that if the drug is removed, the removal will have consequences that must be planned for.

Addiction

Addiction is a different phenomenon entirely. It describes a pattern of compulsive substance use in the face of harm, characterised by loss of control over use, cravings, continued use despite adverse consequences, and, in most modern definitions, changes to the brain's reward circuitry.

Physical dependence is one possible component of addiction, but by itself it is not addiction. A person can be physically dependent on a substance without being addicted to it: think of the person who has taken their blood pressure medication for twenty years and would prefer not to take it, but takes it because their doctor has told them the alternative is a stroke. A person can also be addicted to a substance without being profoundly physically dependent, particularly early in the addiction process.

The relevant fact for our purposes is that antidepressants do not, in the vast majority of cases, produce addiction. Patients on antidepressants do not typically escalate the dose in search of a euphoric effect. They do not typically crave the drug in the way people crave drugs of abuse. They do not typically report loss of control over their use. What they do report, when the dose is reduced or the drug is stopped, is a withdrawal syndrome, which is a signal of physical dependence, not of addiction.

This distinction matters because a person told they are "addicted" to their antidepressant may internalise the label in a way that produces shame and confusion. It matters equally because a prescriber who uses the word addiction to describe a physically dependent patient is loading a diagnosis that does not fit and that may distort the treatment plan.

If you have ever been told by a healthcare worker that you have become "addicted" to your antidepressant, it may be worth a gentle correction. The current, accurate language is that you have developed physical dependence, which is an expected consequence of long-term use, and which is a thing to plan around rather than a thing to be ashamed of.

Withdrawal

Withdrawal is the collection of symptoms that emerges when a substance to which the body has become physically dependent is reduced or removed faster than the body can compensate. It is a physiological event. It has a characteristic timing (often beginning within days of a dose change), a characteristic pattern (often including physical, sensory, and mood symptoms that were not present before the drug was introduced), and a characteristic response to reinstatement (often improving within days when the previous dose is resumed).

For decades, the medical literature used the phrase "discontinuation syndrome" to describe what happens when antidepressants are stopped. The intent behind this phrase was reasonable at the time: to distinguish antidepressant-associated symptoms from the withdrawal syndromes seen with drugs of abuse, and to reassure patients that they were not "addicted" in the pejorative sense. In practice, however, the term "discontinuation syndrome" ended up minimising the phenomenon. It sounded neutral and mild. It suggested a passing inconvenience rather than a physiological event that could last weeks or months. It made it easier for clinicians to dismiss patient reports and easier for patients to feel they were exaggerating.

The current preferred term in the research literature is withdrawal. Not because it is dramatic, but because it is accurate. What happens when you stop a substance to which your body has become adapted is withdrawal, whether the substance is a benzodiazepine, an opioid, an antidepressant, or caffeine.

You will find, if you read across the recent literature, that many clinicians still use "discontinuation syndrome". Do not fight the word with your prescriber. Simply know that what you are experiencing has a name, and that the name has a documented history in the literature stretching back to at least the mid-1990s.

Relapse

Relapse is the return of the original condition that the drug was treating. If you started sertraline for major depression, relapse means the depression coming back. If you started paroxetine for panic disorder, relapse means the panic returning.

Relapse is real, and any book that pretends otherwise is doing you a disservice. Some people who come off their antidepressant will find, after weeks or months of stable functioning, that the condition they originally had returns. When that happens, restarting or trying a different treatment is often the sensible choice.

The problem is that withdrawal and relapse can, on the surface, look similar. Both may involve low mood, anxiety, sleep disturbance, or fatigue. Both may emerge in the weeks following a dose reduction. This is the source of an enormous amount of miscommunication in prescribing offices.

The difference is not in the label of the symptom. It is in the pattern, the timing, and the response to reinstatement.

Withdrawal characteristically begins within days of a dose change, involves physical or sensory symptoms that were not part of the original condition (brain zaps, gait instability, sensory changes, sudden nausea), and improves within days if the previous dose is resumed.

Relapse characteristically emerges over weeks to months after the drug has been stopped or stabilised at a much lower dose, resembles the original condition rather than a new symptom cluster, and does not respond quickly to a small reinstatement.

Chapter 11 will walk you through this distinction in detail, with a decision aid you can bring to a prescriber appointment. For now, hold this: the same feeling, on a Monday two days after cutting your dose in half, and on a Monday ten weeks after finishing the taper, is quite likely to mean two different things.

> **Important Point:** *Withdrawal is a signal about what your nervous system is doing while it re-adapts. Relapse is a signal about the underlying condition. They call for different responses, and the response you choose in the first two weeks of a difficult taper will shape everything that comes after.*

Why this all keeps getting mixed up

If the distinction is this important, why do prescribers and patients keep confusing the four words?

Part of the answer is historical. For most of the past three decades, patients who reported severe or prolonged symptoms after stopping an antidepressant were dismissed. The framing at the time was that antidepressants did not produce dependence in any meaningful sense, that any post-discontinuation symptoms were probably relapse, and that persistent symptoms were probably somatic manifestations of an anxious disposition. Under that framing, there was no need to distinguish withdrawal from relapse, because in effect there was no such thing as antidepressant withdrawal. It was all relapse, or it was all somatic.

Part of the answer is training. Medical schools and psychiatry residencies teach a great deal about starting antidepressants and comparatively little about stopping them. A newly qualified doctor is often more comfortable with the language of prescribing than with the language of tapering. Withdrawal is not routinely covered in the same detail as, say, the side effect profile of the drug at initiation.

Part of the answer is time. A ten-minute appointment does not lend itself to careful language. If a patient reports feeling anxious after a dose reduction, and the prescriber has three minutes to make a decision, restarting the drug is the safe, familiar choice. Distinguishing withdrawal from relapse takes a slower, more attentive conversation than the calendar usually allows.

Part of the answer is the drug companies. In the mid-1990s, several manufacturers actively pushed the term "discontinuation syndrome" as a softer alternative to "withdrawal", specifically because "withdrawal" carried connotations of substance dependence that were commercially unhelpful. Documents from that period are now in the public record. This is not a conspiracy claim; it is a documented fact of pharmaceutical marketing history that has left a small linguistic residue in every prescribing guideline of the era.

None of this is your problem to solve. It is background so that when you notice your prescriber reaching for one of these words in a way that does not fit your situation, you can respectfully say,

"I hear you calling it that. Could we look at whether it might be one of the other terms instead?"

Cashel's example

Cashel was on venlafaxine for eight years when he tried, at his GP's suggestion, to come off over four weeks. Two days after his final dose, he became so dizzy he could not drive. He returned to the surgery, where a locum GP looked at his history and said, "You know, some people just do better on medication. It sounds like the depression is coming back."

Cashel, who was a careful reader and had been keeping a symptom log at his wife's suggestion, said, "I don't feel depressed. I feel like I am inside a washing machine. I have brain zaps every time I move my eyes. I have never felt this before, including when I first came in for the depression."

The locum, to her credit, paused. Then she said, "That does sound different. What do you think is going on?"

Cashel said, "I think I came off it too fast."

She said, "That would fit with what you are describing. Let's put you back on 37.5 mg and see how you are in a week."

Within four days, the dizziness had settled and the brain zaps had stopped. Cashel and the locum agreed to plan a much slower taper this time, over eighteen months, using the methods described in Chapter 8.

The reason that appointment went well was that Cashel had the language. He did not tell the locum she was wrong. He described what he was experiencing accurately, in language that pointed to withdrawal rather than to relapse, and he offered his own interpretation. The locum, given a real description rather than a label, was able to think again.

That is what precise language buys you.

The Named Principle of this chapter: dependence is not addiction, withdrawal is not relapse, and calling any of the four by the wrong name will change the plan in the wrong direction.

In the next chapter, we will look at why standard tapers so often fail, and what "hyperbolic tapering" actually means, in language that does not require a pharmacology degree.

Chapter 3: Why Slow Tapers Still Fail

Ephie had done everything right. She had asked her psychiatrist for a slow taper, and her psychiatrist had agreed. She was on 20 mg of paroxetine. They had planned to reduce by 5 mg every three weeks. Twenty to fifteen, fifteen to ten, ten to five, five to zero, over about three months. This was, in the language of most prescribing guidelines, a slow taper. It was slower than a great many people were offered.

The first two reductions went well. She had a few days of mild lightheadedness after each one, but it settled within a week and she was ready for the next step. Then she cut from 10 mg to 5 mg. Two days later she felt as though the floor was moving. Her sleep collapsed. Brain zaps started every time she turned her head. She held at 5 mg, hoping it would settle. It did not. After ten days she gave up, went back to 10 mg, and told her psychiatrist she could not do it.

She could not understand what had gone wrong. She had reduced by 5 mg each time. Each reduction was the same size in milligrams. Why had the last cut felt like a different order of magnitude?

The answer to Ephie's question is the single most useful piece of pharmacology in this book, and it is the reason the older tapering advice fails so often even when it looks careful on paper.

The receptor curve, in plain English

Imagine a room with a window and a set of blinds. The blinds have twenty slats. When the blinds are fully open, all twenty slats let in light, and the room is bright. When you close the blinds, you close all twenty slats.

Now imagine you are trying to dim the room gradually. You start by closing one slat. The room is very slightly less bright. You close another slat. Again, very slightly less bright. You keep going. By the time you have closed ten slats, the room is noticeably dimmer, but not enormously so, because ten slats are still open and light is coming through them.

Then you close another slat. The room gets a bit darker. Another. And another. And then something interesting happens. You close the eighteenth slat, and the room becomes noticeably darker in a way that the earlier closings did not produce. You close the nineteenth, and now you are close to darkness. You close the twentieth, and you are in the dark.

The last few slats you close produced a much bigger change in the light in the room than the first few slats. Not because those slats were bigger. Not because you were doing anything differently. It is simply that when a lot of slats are already open, closing one more makes almost no difference; when almost none are open, closing the last one is the difference between visible and not.

This is roughly how antidepressant receptor occupancy works. When you start an SSRI at a therapeutic dose, you are, in effect, closing most of the slats. Almost all of the serotonin transporter is occupied by the drug. That is why the effect at the receptor is close to maximal. Now imagine reducing the dose. From 20 mg to 10 mg of, say, citalopram, you have not halved the effect at the receptor. You have gone from perhaps 80% occupancy to perhaps 75% occupancy. The room is still nearly as dark. But when you go from 5 mg to 2.5 mg, you may be dropping from perhaps 60% occupancy to perhaps 40%. That is a much bigger change in what the receptor is actually experiencing.

This is why the last few milligrams of a taper are almost always the hardest, and why Ephie's 10-to-5 cut felt worse than her 20-to-15.

The hyperbolic curve, drawn on paper

If you were to plot dose on the horizontal axis and receptor occupancy on the vertical axis, the resulting line would not be straight. It would curve steeply upward from zero, then flatten out as it approached the top. The technical name for this shape is hyperbolic, from the geometric family of curves. In practical terms, what the curve tells you is that equal reductions in milligrams do not produce equal reductions in effect at the receptor.

The implication for tapering is straightforward, and it is the entire foundation of what is now called hyperbolic tapering.

To produce equal reductions in effect at the receptor, your reductions in milligrams must get smaller as the dose gets smaller. At the top of the dose range, you can reduce by relatively large milligram amounts and produce only small changes at the receptor. Near the bottom of the dose range, you must reduce by very small milligram amounts to avoid producing large changes at the receptor.

Put another way: a taper that looks linear on paper (20, 15, 10, 5, 0) is not linear in what it is doing to your nervous system. Its steps get bigger and bigger in effect as it goes on. What looks like a gentle glide is actually accelerating downwards into a cliff at the end.

A hyperbolic taper looks different on paper. It might be something like 20, 15, 11, 7.5, 5, 3.5, 2.5, 1.75, 1.25, 0.75, 0.5, 0.3, 0.2, 0.1, 0. On paper it looks slow and fiddly. In practice, at the receptor, each step is producing a roughly similar change.

> **Important Point:** *Do not judge a taper by how many milligrams you are dropping. Judge it by how much of the receptor you are freeing up in each step. Late-stage steps that look small in milligrams are often the biggest steps of the whole taper in terms of what they are doing to your brain.*

Why the older advice was wrong, without anyone being wicked

Most of the older advice, the "reduce by 25% and stop after four weeks" guidance you will still see in some clinical settings, was written in an era when this receptor-curve understanding was not yet available. It was not that the people writing the guidance were careless. They were working with the pharmacology that had been established at typical therapeutic doses. Nobody had really looked at what happens at low doses in enough detail to notice that the curve was steep there.

Two things changed in the past decade. First, positron emission tomography imaging studies, which allow researchers to look directly at receptor occupancy in living human brains, produced dose-occupancy curves for several common antidepressants that all showed the same hyperbolic shape. Second, patient reports on peer support forums began to consistently describe the same pattern: the last few milligrams were always the hardest. When Horowitz and Taylor put these two lines of evidence together in a 2019 paper in The Lancet Psychiatry, the field started to shift, and by 2024 the concept of hyperbolic tapering was central to the leading deprescribing guidance published anywhere.

You should not need to know any of this history to plan a taper. But it explains why, if your prescriber is younger than forty or specialises in psychopharmacology, they are more likely to have encountered the hyperbolic model in training, and why, if your prescriber trained in the 1990s and does not specialise in this area, you may need to bring them the reasoning politely. Chapter 14 gives you scripts for that conversation.

What a hyperbolic taper looks like in practice

There are two ways a hyperbolic taper is usually structured, and you will encounter both in the drug-specific chapters that follow.

The first way is proportional reduction. Instead of reducing by a fixed number of milligrams each time (which produces linear cuts and non-linear effect), you reduce by a fixed proportion of the current dose. A common choice is 10% of the current dose per reduction. If you are on 20 mg, your first cut is to 18 mg. From 18, your next cut is to 16.2 mg. And so on. In practice, once the doses get small enough, this produces reductions of a milligram or a fraction of a milligram at a time.

The second way is example schedules. Researchers have worked out approximate step-down sequences that produce roughly equal reductions in receptor occupancy for each of the common antidepressants. Rather than requiring the patient to do the maths themselves, these give a series of doses. For citalopram, the sequence might look something like 20, 15, 10, 6, 4, 2.5, 1.5, 1, 0.5, 0, with time held at each step. For paroxetine, sertraline, and each of the other drugs, the numbers are different, but the shape is the same.

Both approaches produce the same underlying pattern: gentler in real effect at the top, patient and small at the bottom.

You will not need to invent your own schedule. Chapters 7, 8, and 9 give example schedules for each of the drugs this book covers. What you need to take from this chapter is the mental model that makes the schedules make sense.

How long does a taper actually take, then

This is the question everyone wants answered, and it does not have a single answer. The honest range is roughly this.

For a person who has been on a low or moderate dose of an SSRI for a year or less, a taper over three to six months is often manageable, sometimes shorter. For a person who has been on a moderate to high dose for several years, a taper over six to twelve months is common. For a person who has been on a difficult drug (paroxetine, venlafaxine, duloxetine) for many years, tapers of twelve to twenty-four months are not unusual, and some patients take longer.

If those numbers feel long, hold this: the alternative for many long-term users is not a shorter taper but a failed taper. A twelve-month taper that succeeds is much shorter than a four-week taper that fails, ends in reinstatement, and is not attempted again for another five years.

You are not tapering to a deadline. You are tapering to zero, at whatever pace your nervous system can follow.

Ephie's revised plan

When Ephie and her psychiatrist looked at what had happened, they realised that her 5 mg reductions had been reasonable at the top of her dose range and had become far too large at the bottom. Her paroxetine schedule was rewritten. From 20 mg, she went to 15, then to 12, then to 10, then to 8, then to 6.5, then to 5, then to 4, then to 3, then to 2.25, then to 1.5, then to 1, then to 0.5, then to 0. Each step was held for at least four weeks before the next reduction, longer if symptoms did not fully settle. To get the small doses, she used a licensed liquid formulation of paroxetine, which we will return to in Chapter 6.

The whole taper took her a little over eighteen months. She had one bad month, around 4 mg, which surprised her. She held for eight weeks before the next step, and it settled. She reached zero the week of her son's ninth birthday.

She said, later, "I could not believe how small the last cuts were. Half a milligram to zero. It felt ridiculous. But when I look back, I think if I had done that jump at four weeks in, I would have lost the whole thing."

She is right, and the reason she is right is the shape of the curve.

The Key Takeaway of this chapter: reductions must get smaller in milligrams as the dose gets smaller, because equal steps in milligrams are not equal steps at the receptor.

In the next chapter, we will look at whether now is the right time for you to start, because a good plan attempted at the wrong moment often turns into a lost taper. Readiness matters, and it is worth taking a chapter to check.

Chapter 4: Are You Ready, and Is Now the Right Time

There is a version of this book I did not write, in which every chapter urges you toward the door, and readiness is a matter of getting past your reluctance. That book would sell better. It would also do harm, because coming off an antidepressant at the wrong time, in the wrong life circumstances, with the wrong support around you, is one of the most reliable ways to end up with a failed taper and a longer stretch on the drug than you had planned for.

Readiness is not a mystical quality. It is a set of practical conditions that make a taper more likely to succeed. This chapter walks you through those conditions and helps you decide whether to start now, start soon with some preparatory changes, or deliberately postpone.

Why timing matters this much

A taper is a controlled destabilisation of a system that has adapted to a drug. Even when it goes well, it demands something from the person doing it. Sleep may be less reliable for a stretch. Mood may be a bit more variable. Concentration may be a bit patchier. Physical energy may dip. These effects are usually manageable, and they usually resolve. But they are not zero, and they land on top of whatever else is happening in your life at the same time.

A person tapering during a stable period, with reasonable sleep, a job that permits some flexibility, at least one supportive person at home, and a prescriber willing to help, is doing something quite different from a person tapering while working night shifts, going through a divorce, sleeping four hours a night, and being told by their GP that antidepressant withdrawal is not a real thing.

The first person has room to absorb the taper. The second person does not.

The good news is that room is a matter of adjustment. Some readers will read this chapter and realise they are ready. Some will realise they need to sort out one or two things first. Some will realise that six months from now would be a much better time, and that using those six months to prepare will make the actual taper faster and safer when they do start.

There is no prize for starting today.

Life stability

The first cluster of readiness questions is about the shape of your life right now.

Are you in stable housing? Not perfect housing, not permanent housing, but housing that is not going to change in the next few months. Moving house during a taper is a common way to add unnecessary stress at the exact wrong time.

Is your primary relationship stable? Again, not perfect, not necessarily happy, but not in acute crisis. If you are in the middle of a separation, a breakup, or a serious relationship crisis, that is a bad moment to also destabilise your neurochemistry. If the relationship crisis is expected to resolve within a defined timeframe, wait until it does.

Are you working, and if so, is the work manageable? Some tapers can be done during ordinary work. Others require the person to reduce hours or take some form of leave during the harder stretches. If you are self-employed, or on a zero-hours contract, or working night shifts, or in a role that punishes any drop in performance, factor this into your planning.

Is there a birth, a death, or a major life transition coming in the next few months? Weddings, funerals, house moves, first babies, second babies, new jobs, moves abroad. Any of these will consume energy you might need for the taper.

None of these are absolute barriers. People successfully taper through busy periods. But if two or three of these questions produce difficult answers, that is worth noticing.

Support around you

The second cluster of questions is about who you have.

Is there at least one person in your household or your immediate life who understands what you are doing and can support you? This does not have to be a therapist or a doctor. It can be a partner, a sibling, a close friend. What matters is that when you have a bad day, there is someone to whom you can say "I am having a rough patch, it is probably the taper, I am not going back on the drug, I just need to say it out loud."

Is your prescriber willing to work with you on a slower taper than the standard advice? If the answer is yes, that is a significant asset. If the answer is not yet, Chapter 14 has scripts for the conversation you need to have. If the answer is a hard no and the prescriber will not budge, you may need to change prescribers before you begin.

Do you have access to a pharmacy that can help with the formulations you will need? For readers on standard doses of common SSRIs, ordinary pharmacies can usually meet the need. For readers on venlafaxine or paroxetine planning to reduce below the smallest pill dose, access to a compounding pharmacy or a licensed liquid can be the difference between a completable taper and a stuck one.

Do you have anyone to whom you can turn if things get worse rather than better? This does not have to be crisis-level; it might just be someone you trust who can hear "I am worried I made the wrong call" and help you think it through.

Your reasons for wanting to come off

The third cluster is about what is bringing you to this decision.

The most durable reasons for coming off are reasons that will still make sense to you in six months if the taper is being difficult. Something like: I have been on this drug for eight years and I want to know what my emotional baseline actually is; I am experiencing a side effect that outweighs the benefit for me; I am planning a pregnancy and want to be off before conception; the reason I started the drug is no longer part of my life, and I want to see whether the drug is still needed.

Less durable reasons are ones that may not survive the first difficult month. Something like: my partner thinks I should not need this; I saw a documentary that made me nervous about long-term use; someone I know had a bad experience and now I am worried.

None of the less durable reasons is invalid, but they may not be robust enough to carry you through a hard patch. If your reason for coming off is external, it may help to talk it through with a therapist or a trusted person before you start, and to check whether there is an underlying reason of your own that you have not yet named.

The choice of a lower dose rather than zero

Not every taper needs to end at zero. Some patients do very well on a partial taper, coming down to a lower long-term dose that gives them fewer side effects while still providing meaningful benefit.

If your reason for coming off is that a specific side effect is bothering you, and if that side effect tends to be dose-related, a partial taper is often worth considering as an initial goal. You can always continue to zero later if you want to. What you gain by aiming lower first is a clearer picture of whether the side effect resolves at the reduced dose, and whether the benefit you get from the drug is preserved. Some people discover, in the course of a partial taper, that they feel best on a much lower dose than they were originally prescribed and choose to stay there. That is a legitimate outcome.

The book will assume that your goal is zero unless you say otherwise, but the schedules can be adapted to stop at any dose you and your prescriber agree on.

Your readiness scoresheet

Take a moment now to answer the following, honestly.

Housing is stable for at least the next six months: yes, no, uncertain.

Primary relationship is not in acute crisis: yes, no, uncertain.

Work is manageable, or I can reduce or adjust work if needed: yes, no, uncertain.

No major life transitions expected in the next six months: yes, no, uncertain.

At least one person in my life understands what I am doing: yes, no, uncertain.

My prescriber is willing to support a slow taper: yes, no, uncertain.

I have pharmacy access for the formulations I will need: yes, no, uncertain, do not yet know what I will need.

My reason for coming off is one I will still hold in six months: yes, no, uncertain.

I have a clear goal (zero, or a specific lower dose): yes, no, uncertain.

I am not currently in a mental health crisis: yes, no, uncertain.

If you have answered yes to eight or more of these, you are probably ready to plan and start.

If you have answered yes to five to seven, you are probably ready to plan, but you have one or two conditions to sort out before you begin. Use the next few weeks or months to sort them out.

If you have answered yes to fewer than five, please consider deliberately postponing. Set a review date, three or six months from now, and use the time to work on the conditions that were not yet met. That review date is not a failure. It is a plan with a longer preface.

> **Important Point:** *A taper delayed until conditions are right is not a taper avoided. It is a taper that is more likely to succeed.*

When postponing is the harder call

There is a group of readers for whom postponing feels like giving in. You have decided you want to come off, and to be told to wait is to be told that the decision does not belong to you.

The decision does belong to you. The reason to postpone is not that you should not be doing this. The reason to postpone is that starting a difficult process now, when the conditions are working against you, has a higher probability of ending in a return to the drug at the same dose or a higher one than you are on now. Postponing is a strategic choice, not a moral one.

There is also a group of readers for whom postponing is a way of never starting. If you notice yourself using the readiness questions as a way to keep the taper permanently in the future, that is worth noticing too. Some people benefit from setting a start date at the top of a diary, six months out, and treating the intervening period as active preparation rather than as an extension of doing nothing.

If you are unsure which group you are in, that is a good conversation to have with a therapist, if you have one, or with a trusted person if you do not.

Auguste's postponement

Auguste was 34 and had been on sertraline for six years. He came in around Christmas, having decided he wanted to come off. He was also, at the same time, three months into a demanding new job, planning to propose to his girlfriend, and preparing to fly home to see his parents for the first time in two years.

We went through the readiness questions. Yes to housing, yes to relationship stability, yes to prescriber willingness, no to work being manageable during the first six months of the new role, no to no transitions, yes to reason, yes to support, unsure to pharmacy access because he was not sure of his goal dose. Six yeses, two nos, one unsure.

I told him he was probably ready to plan, but that I would recommend setting the start date for June, six months out, and using the intervening months to consolidate the new job, get engaged, see his parents, and pick a prescriber he trusted for the taper itself. He did not want to hear this. He said he had been thinking about it for a year.

He also said, before he left, that he trusted the reasoning even though he did not like it.

He came back in May, ready to plan the taper properly. He was engaged, settled in the job, and the visit home had gone well. His nervous system, when it came time for the first reduction, had room to absorb it. His taper took about ten months and was, in his description, difficult but never frightening.

If we had started in January, it might have been quite a different story.

The Named Principle of this chapter: readiness is not a mood, it is a set of conditions, and the conditions can be built.

In the next chapter, we will look at how to turn all this preparation into a written taper plan you can bring to your prescriber.

Chapter 5: Building Your Taper Plan

Zowie had been on 50 mg of sertraline for four years. She had done Chapter 4's readiness check and come out on the safe side of it. She had spoken to her GP, who had agreed to a slower taper than the standard four-week reduction. She had a supportive partner, a job she could adjust if needed, and a clear reason for wanting to come off (she felt she had lost her ability to cry, and she wanted it back).

She sat down at her kitchen table and pulled out a notebook. She wrote at the top of the page: My Taper Plan. And then she did not know what to write next.

This is where most people arrive after they have decided to start. The principles make sense. The readiness questions have been answered. The prescriber is on side. And yet drawing up the actual plan feels like standing at the base of a mountain without a map.

This chapter is the map. By the end, you will have a draft plan you can adapt with your prescriber. The plan will not be permanent (real tapers change as they go), but it will be a starting document that reflects the pharmacology of your specific drug, your specific life circumstances, and your specific goal.

The five decisions your plan has to make

Every taper plan is built from five decisions. Once you have made these, you have a plan.

The first decision is your initial reduction size. This is the size of the first cut, expressed as a percentage of your current dose.

The second decision is your reduction interval. This is the length of time you will hold each new dose before making the next reduction.

The third decision is your reduction pattern. This is whether you will use fixed-percentage cuts (each step is the same percentage of the current dose) or a pre-worked example schedule (a table of specific doses to step through).

The fourth decision is your goal. This is the dose you are aiming to reach. For most readers this is zero, but a partial taper to a lower long-term dose is also legitimate.

The fifth decision is your review points. These are the dates in the plan where you will pause, take stock, and either continue or adjust.

These five decisions are what your plan is. Everything else is detail.

Decision one: initial reduction size

The three most common starting reduction sizes in current use are 25%, 10%, and 5% of the current dose.

A 25% initial reduction is appropriate for people who have been on a low dose of a well-tolerated drug for a short time (weeks to a few months), have no history of difficult tapers, and are on a drug with a long half-life. In practice, this is a minority of readers of this book.

A 10% initial reduction is a common middle-ground choice. It is often used as a starting point for readers who have been on a moderate dose for months to a few years, have not attempted a taper before, and are on a drug of average difficulty. Most SSRI tapers in this book will start here.

A 5% initial reduction is used for readers who have been on a drug for many years, have attempted a taper before that produced significant withdrawal, or are on a drug of known difficulty (paroxetine, venlafaxine, duloxetine). It is also used when the person has a highly sensitive nervous system by history, meaning that they tend to be more responsive than average to small changes in medication generally.

The general rule is: it is safer to start too small and speed up if you tolerate it well than to start too large and back off. The consequences of starting too small are a slightly longer overall taper. The consequences of starting too large are a destabilised nervous system, a lost month, and often a lost taper.

If in doubt, start with 10%. If you have a history of difficult tapers or you are on venlafaxine or paroxetine, start with 5%. If you are on fluoxetine after less than a year, 25% is often reasonable.

Decision two: reduction interval

The most common interval between reductions is two to four weeks. The interval you choose depends on how long the drug takes to reach a new steady state at each new dose, and on how long you want to hold at that new state before deciding whether it is stable.

For drugs with short half-lives (venlafaxine, paroxetine), a new steady state is reached quickly, but the nervous system may need longer to settle. Two to four weeks is a common minimum.

For drugs with long half-lives (fluoxetine, and to a lesser extent sertraline and citalopram), the drug takes several weeks to reach a new steady state, and the interval between reductions may need to be at least four weeks to see the true effect of the reduction.

For mirtazapine and trazodone, where the primary reason to hold is to give sleep architecture time to stabilise, three to four weeks per step is often needed.

You are not looking for the interval that finishes the taper fastest. You are looking for the interval that lets you know, before you make the next cut, whether the previous cut has settled.

> **Important Point:** *A dose reduction is only worth counting as done when the symptoms it produced have fully settled. If you cut again while still symptomatic, you are stacking two reductions on top of a nervous system that has not caught up with the first one, and you will pay for it.*

Decision three: pattern

The choice between fixed-percentage cuts and an example schedule comes down to what suits your temperament and what your pharmacist and prescriber can support.

Fixed-percentage cuts are transparent and mathematically consistent. You start on your current dose, cut by 10%, hold, cut by another 10% of the new dose, hold, and so on. The advantage is that you can always work out the next dose yourself, and the pattern will naturally produce hyperbolic behaviour (each cut is smaller in absolute terms than the last). The disadvantage is that you need a formulation that lets you actually deliver the small doses this produces late in the taper.

Example schedules are pre-worked tables developed by researchers for specific drugs. For each of the drugs in this book, Chapters 7, 8, and 9 give one such table. The advantage is that you can hand the table to your prescriber and pharmacist and simply follow it. The disadvantage is less flexibility if your body wants to move faster or slower than the table anticipates.

Many people use a hybrid: they start with an example schedule, and then move to fixed-percentage cuts once they are used to the pattern.

Decision four: goal

Zero is the default assumption for most readers. Some readers will choose a lower long-term dose. A small number will decide, partway through the taper, to stop the taper at a lower dose and hold there. All of these are legitimate outcomes.

Write down your goal now, in one sentence. "I want to come off entirely" or "I want to reduce to 5 mg and hold there for a year and reassess" or "I want to see if I can get to zero and if not I want to be on the lowest dose that keeps the depression manageable". Whatever your goal is, name it.

You can change your goal later. But naming it now gives your plan a shape, and it gives you a reference point when things get difficult.

Decision five: review points

Every taper plan should have built-in review points. These are dates on which you will pause and make a deliberate assessment: is this working, is this on track, do I need to adjust, do I need to slow down, do I need to speak to my prescriber?

For most tapers, a review point every three months is a sensible minimum. You may also want to schedule a review after any particularly difficult reduction, and after any planned hold that lasted longer than expected.

Review points are not decision points where you must continue or stop. They are simply moments where you slow down and look at the plan with fresh eyes. Most of the time, you will decide to continue. Occasionally, you will decide to change something, and that is what the review points are for.

Zowie's draft plan

Zowie's plan, when she finished it that evening at her kitchen table, looked like this.

Drug: sertraline. Current dose: 50 mg. Duration of use: four years. Prior tapers: none. Goal: zero, over roughly twelve to eighteen months, revising as needed.

Initial reduction size: 10% of current dose.

Reduction interval: four weeks minimum, longer if not settled.

Pattern: fixed-percentage cuts, using a spreadsheet she would build (she was that kind of person), with the first several doses being 50, 45, 40, 36, 32, 28, 25, 22, 20, and continuing down in a similar pattern until she could no longer use whole-tablet doses. At that point she planned to switch to sertraline liquid to reach doses below 25 mg with precision.

Review points: at three months, at six months, at nine months, and after any hold longer than six weeks.

That draft, on a single sheet of paper, was her taper plan.

She took it to her GP the following week. Her GP looked at it, made two adjustments (she wanted a slightly longer initial interval, and she wanted an in-person check at the six-week mark rather than three months), and they signed off on the revised version. The whole conversation took ten minutes.

What if your prescriber wants a different plan

You may go to your appointment with a draft like Zowie's, and your prescriber may propose changes. Most of the time, these will be sensible. Sometimes they will be a shift back toward the older, faster tapering advice. This is where the language you learned in Chapter 2, and the science you learned in Chapter 3, and the scripts you will meet in Chapter 14, become useful.

The general principle is that this is a negotiation, not a submission. Your prescriber knows things you do not (about your history, about drug interactions, about local pharmacy options).

You know things they do not (about how your body has responded in the past to changes, about what you can absorb in your life right now, about what you want the outcome to be). A good plan is drawn up between the two of you.

If your prescriber is not willing to work with a slower plan under any circumstances, you have a decision to make. Sometimes the answer is to try, and see how the first reduction goes. Sometimes the answer is to find a different prescriber. Neither is wrong. What is wrong is to accept a plan you already know is too fast for you and then blame yourself when it fails.

The taper log

Every plan needs a log alongside it. You will start keeping this log the day before your first reduction, and you will keep it going all the way to zero.

The log has three functions. First, it lets you see patterns in your symptoms across time, patterns that would be invisible if you were only remembering the last two days. Second, it gives your prescriber real data to work with when you have appointments. Third, it protects you from the two most common cognitive errors during a taper: catastrophising a bad day as evidence that the whole plan is failing, and minimising a genuine trend as "just a bad patch".

The log does not have to be complicated. A daily entry that captures: date, current dose, sleep quality on a one-to-five scale, mood on a one-to-five scale, physical symptoms (any of the list from Chapter 10), and one line on how the day went. Some people prefer a spreadsheet. Some prefer a paper diary. Some use an app. The format matters less than the habit.

You will thank yourself for keeping this log by around week eight, when you have a bad day and can look back and see that you had a similar day four weeks ago and it passed.

The Key Takeaway of this chapter: a plan on paper is not a taper, but a taper without a plan on paper is chaos with a receipt.

In the next chapter, we will look at the formulation problem: how to actually deliver the small doses your plan calls for when your pharmacy only stocks whole tablets.

Chapter 6: Getting the Doses You Need

Lorcan needed to reduce his venlafaxine from 37.5 mg to 30 mg. That was his next planned step. His pharmacy stocked 37.5 mg and 75 mg capsules. Nothing in between. When he asked for smaller doses, the pharmacist told him there was no smaller strength manufactured. When he asked for a liquid, the pharmacist told him none was licensed in his country. When he went back to his GP and asked what to do, his GP said, "Just cut them in half."

Lorcan tried to cut a 37.5 mg venlafaxine capsule in half. What he found, when he opened the capsule, was that it did not contain a homogenous white powder that could be halved. It contained hundreds of tiny beads. Halving the capsule did not halve the dose. It scattered beads across his kitchen counter.

This is where more tapers stall than at any other point. The plan on paper calls for a dose that does not exist as a manufactured pill. The pharmacy cannot supply it. The prescriber does not know how to prescribe it. The patient is left with a choice between doing a jump that is too large and giving up.

This chapter is about the ways around that problem. Some of them are elegant, some are fiddly, and one or two involve maths. All of them are ways to get the specific dose your plan calls for, when the standard supply chain will not give it to you.

Licensed liquid formulations

The simplest solution, when it is available, is a licensed liquid formulation of your drug. A licensed liquid means that the manufacturer has produced and sold a liquid version of the medication, complete with a specific concentration, that your prescriber can write a prescription for and your pharmacy can dispense.

Not every antidepressant has a licensed liquid form, and availability varies by country. In the UK, at the time of writing, licensed liquids exist for citalopram, escitalopram, fluoxetine, paroxetine, sertraline (varying availability), and mirtazapine (as an oro-dispersible tablet, though this is not the same as a true liquid). In the United States, availability is broader for some drugs and narrower for others. In Australia and Canada, it varies again.

The advantage of a licensed liquid is that it comes with a manufacturer-tested concentration, so a specific volume of liquid delivers a specific dose reliably. The disadvantage is that not all liquids are widely stocked, some are more expensive than the tablet or capsule form, and some pharmacists will need to order them in.

The way to get one is straightforward. Your prescriber writes a prescription for the liquid form, at the concentration and volume you agree on. Your pharmacist orders it in if they do not stock it. You measure out your dose using a syringe (usually supplied with the liquid) rather than counting pills.

If you are going to reduce below the smallest tablet dose of your drug, and if a licensed liquid exists for it, this is almost always the easiest route. Chapter 14 has a specific script for asking your prescriber for a liquid switch.

Compounding pharmacies

When a licensed liquid does not exist, or when it exists but at a concentration that does not match your needs, a compounding pharmacy can often help.

A compounding pharmacy is a pharmacy that prepares medications individually, to a specific formulation, rather than dispensing pre-manufactured tablets. Compounding pharmacies can prepare liquid versions of medications for which no licensed liquid exists, at whatever concentration you and your prescriber specify. They can also prepare specific low-dose tablets or capsules.

Not every country regulates compounding pharmacies the same way, and the exact process varies. In some countries, any licensed pharmacy can compound; in others, only specific compounding pharmacies do so. Your prescriber will usually know local options, or your regular pharmacy will be able to refer you.

The advantage of compounded formulations is flexibility: you can, in principle, get any dose you need. The disadvantages are cost (compounded medications are usually more expensive than manufactured ones and are not always covered by insurance), availability (compounding pharmacies may not be within convenient distance), and shelf life (compounded liquids often have shorter expiry dates than manufactured ones).

If your drug does not have a licensed liquid and you need doses below the smallest manufactured tablet, compounding is often the way to get there. This is particularly relevant for venlafaxine and desvenlafaxine, both of which have limited licensed liquid options in many countries.

Bead counting for capsules

Venlafaxine extended release and duloxetine both come in capsules that contain many small beads. Each bead contains a small amount of the drug, formulated for slow release. In principle, opening the capsule and removing a proportion of the beads reduces the total dose in a controlled way.

The method works like this. You open the capsule carefully over a clean surface. You count the beads (or, for larger doses, weigh them on a fine kitchen scale). You then remove the number of beads corresponding to the reduction you want, and take the remainder.

Suppose your venlafaxine 75 mg capsule contains, roughly, 300 beads. Each bead is worth approximately 0.25 mg. If your plan calls for a 10% reduction, from 75 to 67.5 mg, you would remove roughly 30 beads and take the remaining 270. If you want to reduce by 5%, you would remove 15 beads.

The advantage of this method is that it is cheap, uses the standard manufactured capsule, and can produce very small dose reductions with reasonable precision. The disadvantage is that it is fiddly, requires careful counting or weighing, and works only with capsules that contain beads (not with all extended-release formulations).

You should not use this method without your prescriber's knowledge, and you should not use it with capsules that are not designed to be opened. The beads inside extended-release capsules of venlafaxine and duloxetine are designed to be swallowed with a small amount of soft food if needed, but not all capsules are like this. Ask your pharmacist whether the specific capsule you have is safe to open.

> **Important Point:** *If you are going to use bead counting, use it consistently. Do not switch between bead counting and pill halving mid-taper, because you will introduce dose variability that makes it harder to interpret how you are doing.*

Tapering strips

A tapering strip is a manufactured product in which each day's dose is slightly smaller than the previous day's, packaged in a sequential strip. Instead of manually reducing your dose every few weeks, you take the dose in front of you each day, and it declines according to a pre-calculated schedule.

Tapering strips were developed by researchers at Cinderella Therapeutics in the Netherlands, and their availability is currently uneven. In some European countries, they can be ordered by a prescriber. In others, they are difficult to obtain. In the United States, they are not currently marketed. In the UK, availability has been variable.

The advantage of tapering strips is convenience: the day-to-day reductions are worked out for you, and you do not have to count beads or measure liquid. The disadvantage is availability, cost, and the fact that some strips use a schedule that is faster than the patient's nervous system can tolerate.

If you have access to tapering strips and your prescriber is willing to prescribe them, they can be a useful tool. If you do not, do not spend a lot of energy chasing them. The other methods in this chapter can achieve the same thing.

Pill splitting

The simplest and cheapest method, and the one most likely to be suggested by a prescriber who has not been trained in modern tapering, is pill splitting.

Pill splitting works, up to a point, for tablets that are scored and reasonably homogenous. A citalopram 20 mg tablet, for example, can be split into two 10 mg halves reasonably reliably, using a pill cutter designed for the purpose.

The limits of pill splitting are two. First, most tablets cannot be reliably split into quarters or eighths; the resulting pieces are of variable dose. Second, extended-release formulations cannot be split at all, because splitting them disrupts the release mechanism and can produce a much faster release than the drug was designed for. If your drug is an extended-release preparation, do not split it. If your drug is a capsule, do not attempt to open it unless you have specifically checked that it is designed to be opened.

For the top half of a taper, when you are still working with reductions of 5 mg or more at a time from a moderate-to-high dose, pill splitting can carry you a long way. For the bottom half, it usually cannot, and you will need one of the other methods.

Water titration

Water titration is the practice of dissolving a tablet or the contents of a capsule in a known volume of water, and then taking a specific fraction of that solution to achieve a small dose. It is used at home by some patients, often in combination with a syringe or a graduated measuring cup.

Water titration can work, in principle, for some drugs. It is not safe or accurate for others. Whether a specific tablet dissolves properly in water, whether the drug remains stable in solution, and whether the drug is evenly distributed in the water are all important questions, and the answers vary by drug.

Because of these variables, and because water titration is not a formally approved method for most antidepressants, this book will not give you a specific water titration protocol. If your prescriber is willing to supervise water titration for your specific drug, and if they have looked into whether it is appropriate, that can be a workable method. If you are trying to work it out on your own, you will get more reliable dosing from a licensed liquid or from a compounded liquid, and you should pursue those first.

Cross-tapering to fluoxetine

For some drugs, particularly paroxetine and venlafaxine, one of the historical options for a difficult taper has been to switch to fluoxetine first, and then to taper the fluoxetine. The rationale is that fluoxetine's long half-life means that reducing it is much more forgiving than reducing paroxetine or venlafaxine directly, and the transition to fluoxetine can sometimes bypass the acute withdrawal that a direct taper would produce.

The fluoxetine bridge is not for everyone. It is more helpful for people who have already struggled to reduce their current drug directly. It is less appropriate for people who have not tried a direct taper and might do fine with one. It also does not always work: some patients cross-taper to fluoxetine and still find the fluoxetine taper difficult, though usually less so than the original drug.

If a fluoxetine bridge is being considered, it should be planned with a prescriber who is familiar with it. There are specific dose equivalences (10 mg of paroxetine is roughly equivalent to 20 mg of fluoxetine, and so on) and specific cross-over patterns. This is not a method to attempt without medical guidance.

Chapters 7 and 8 will flag which drugs are candidates for a fluoxetine bridge.

Choosing your formulation approach

You now have six methods in front of you: licensed liquid, compounded liquid, bead counting, tapering strips, pill splitting, water titration, and cross-taper to fluoxetine. That is seven, actually. In practice, most tapers use a combination.

For the top of the taper, when reductions are relatively large in absolute terms, pill splitting or full pills often work.

For the middle of the taper, licensed or compounded liquid is often the cleanest option.

For the bottom of the taper, licensed or compounded liquid becomes essential for most drugs, because the reductions are simply too small to achieve any other way.

For venlafaxine and duloxetine specifically, bead counting is a common approach at the mid-to-bottom of the taper because of the way these capsules are formulated.

For paroxetine and venlafaxine, a fluoxetine bridge is worth considering if the direct taper has already been difficult.

Your job now is to look at your plan from Chapter 5, look at the doses it calls for, and work out which method or combination of methods will let you actually deliver those doses. Then you have the second half of the conversation with your prescriber and pharmacist: not just about the schedule, but about how you will physically achieve each dose.

Lorcan's answer, when he thought about it, was to switch to compounded venlafaxine liquid, at a concentration of 5 mg per ml. That let him measure out any dose he wanted with a 1 ml syringe. His compounding pharmacy was forty minutes away by car, and the liquid was more expensive than the capsules, but for the first time in eighteen months of trying he had a method that would let him actually implement his plan.

The Important Point of this chapter: your plan is only as good as your ability to deliver the doses it calls for. Solve the formulation problem before you make the next cut.

In the next chapter, we turn to the drug-specific schedules for SSRIs.

Chapter 7: Coming Off SSRIs

The SSRI chapter is the longest in this book, because five drugs live here and each of them behaves slightly differently. Read the general section first, then read the section on your specific drug. If you are on more than one antidepressant, focus on the one you plan to reduce first (which should almost always be one drug at a time, not both together).

Every example schedule in this chapter is exactly that: an example. It is not a prescription. Bring the relevant table to your prescriber. Discuss whether the starting reduction size, the interval, and the pattern fit your history. Adjust as needed together.

General principles that apply to all SSRIs

Every SSRI schedule in this chapter follows the same underlying logic. The reductions are hyperbolic in shape, meaning that the milligram size of each cut gets smaller as the dose gets smaller. The intervals between cuts are calibrated to the drug's half-life and to a general principle of giving your nervous system enough time to settle before you ask it to change again. The example schedules assume a moderate-duration user (two to eight years on the drug) at a moderate starting dose. If you have been on the drug for longer, or if your history includes a difficult prior taper, you will typically want smaller cuts held for longer.

The interval between cuts, in every SSRI example schedule, is a minimum of two weeks and typically four weeks. If, at any interval, the symptoms of the previous reduction have not fully settled, you hold at that dose until they do. This is the single most important operating rule of a taper, and it takes precedence over the calendar.

Bupropion, which is sometimes prescribed alongside an SSRI, is not covered in this chapter because it works on a different pharmacology and generally produces a milder withdrawal syndrome. If you are on bupropion together with an SSRI, the current pragmatic advice is to taper the SSRI first, using this chapter, and then the bupropion separately with your prescriber.

Sertraline (Zoloft)

Sertraline has a half-life of around 26 hours. It is commonly prescribed at doses between 25 mg and 200 mg for depression, anxiety, panic disorder, and post-traumatic stress disorder. It is generally regarded as one of the easier SSRIs to taper, though "easier" is relative and does not mean easy.

A licensed liquid form of sertraline exists in some countries at a concentration that allows relatively small doses to be measured. Where it does, this is often the cleanest approach for the second half of the taper.

An example hyperbolic schedule from 50 mg:

Step	Dose (mg)	Time at Dose (weeks, minimum)
Starting	50	4
1	45	4
2	40	4
3	35	4
4	30	4
5	25	4
6	20	4
7	15	4
8	10	4
9	7	4
10	5	4

Step	Dose (mg)	Time at Dose (weeks, minimum)
11	3.5	4
12	2	4
13	1	4
14	0.5	4
15	0	(final)

That schedule spans roughly fourteen months at the minimum-interval assumption. Real tapers often add holds and take longer.

For higher starting doses (100, 150, or 200 mg), the initial steps are proportionally larger and the pattern continues in the same way. For lower starting doses (25 mg or lower), you enter the schedule roughly at step 6 or 7.

Common sertraline withdrawal symptoms include mild dizziness, brain zaps (usually less severe than with paroxetine or venlafaxine), gastrointestinal upset, headaches, and anxiety rebound. Sleep disturbance is possible but is generally less severe than with paroxetine.

Escitalopram (Cipralex, Lexapro)

Escitalopram has a half-life of around 27 to 32 hours. It is commonly prescribed at doses between 5 mg and 20 mg for depression and anxiety. It is generally regarded as one of the more manageable SSRIs to taper, though its withdrawal syndrome can be more marked than sertraline's, particularly for people who have been on it for many years.

A licensed liquid form of escitalopram exists in most markets and is often the easiest way to reach the small doses at the bottom of the taper.

An example hyperbolic schedule from 10 mg:

Step	Dose (mg)	Time at Dose (weeks, minimum)
Starting	10	4
1	9	4
2	8	4
3	7	4
4	6	4
5	5	4
6	4	4
7	3.2	4
8	2.5	4
9	1.75	4
10	1.25	4
11	0.75	4
12	0.5	4
13	0.25	4
14	0	(final)

Common escitalopram withdrawal symptoms include dizziness, brain zaps, sensory changes (particularly light and sound sensitivity), mood volatility, and occasional gastrointestinal upset. The last few milligrams are typically the hardest, which is a pattern you will see repeated across all of the drugs in this chapter.

Citalopram (Celexa, Cipramil)

Citalopram has a half-life of around 35 hours. It is commonly prescribed at doses between 10 mg and 40 mg for depression and anxiety. In many respects it behaves similarly to escitalopram, which is its more selective sister compound, though the tapering schedules are not identical because the dose ranges differ.

A licensed liquid form of citalopram exists in most markets. Where doses smaller than the smallest available tablet are needed, the liquid is often the way to reach them.

An example hyperbolic schedule from 20 mg:

Step	Dose (mg)	Time at Dose (weeks, minimum)
Starting	20	4
1	18	4
2	16	4
3	14	4
4	12	4
5	10	4
6	8	4
7	6	4
8	4.5	4
9	3	4
10	2	4
11	1.5	4
12	1	4
13	0.5	4
14	0	(final)

Common citalopram withdrawal symptoms are similar to those of escitalopram, though for many patients the withdrawal from citalopram is somewhat gentler. If you have never tried a taper before and you are on citalopram at a low or moderate dose, this drug is often one of the more forgiving to reduce.

Fluoxetine (Prozac)

Fluoxetine has, effectively, the longest half-life of any drug in this book. Its parent compound has a half-life of one to three days, and its active metabolite norfluoxetine has a half-life of one to two weeks. In practical terms, this means that after you take a dose of fluoxetine, the drug leaves your system very slowly, and the concentration in your blood is very stable between doses.

This makes fluoxetine substantially easier to taper than the other drugs in this chapter, for two reasons. First, because the drug's own long half-life produces a natural cushioning effect at each dose reduction (the drug is effectively tapering itself for several weeks after each cut). Second, because missed doses do not produce the acute withdrawal that missed doses of the other SSRIs can produce.

Fluoxetine is available as a licensed liquid in most markets.

An example schedule from 20 mg:

Step	Dose (mg)	Time at Dose (weeks, minimum)
Starting	20	4
1	15	4
2	10	6
3	8	6
4	6	6
5	4	6
6	2	6
7	1	6

Step	Dose (mg)	Time at Dose (weeks, minimum)
8	0.5	6
9	0	(final)

Note the longer intervals in the second half of the schedule. This reflects the very long half-life: even after you make a cut, the effect at the receptor continues to decline for several weeks. If you cut again too soon, you may find yourself stacked with cumulative reductions.

Common fluoxetine withdrawal symptoms are typically milder than those from any other drug in this chapter. Some patients report no discernible withdrawal at all. Others report late-emerging symptoms weeks after the final dose, because the drug is only now truly leaving the system.

If you are considering a fluoxetine bridge from another drug, this is the drug you would be bridging to, and your prescriber will be able to work out the equivalent dose.

Paroxetine (Paxil, Seroxat)

Paroxetine is the SSRI with the reputation of being hardest to come off, and the reputation is deserved. Its half-life is around 21 hours, on the short side for an SSRI. It has muscarinic receptor activity that other SSRIs do not have, which produces additional anticholinergic withdrawal symptoms (dry mouth, constipation, blurred vision) that other SSRIs do not typically produce. And its receptor occupancy curve is particularly steep at low doses, meaning that the last few milligrams are especially difficult.

A licensed liquid form of paroxetine exists in most markets, and using it is often essential for a successful taper.

An example hyperbolic schedule from 20 mg, tapered more slowly than the other SSRIs:

Step	Dose (mg)	Time at Dose (weeks, minimum)
Starting	20	4
1	18	4
2	16	4
3	14	4
4	12	4
5	10	4
6	8	4
7	6.5	4
8	5	4
9	4	4
10	3	4
11	2.25	4
12	1.5	4
13	1	4
14	0.5	4
15	0.25	4
16	0	(final)

Real paroxetine tapers frequently take longer than this, particularly at the bottom. Do not be surprised if a cut that looks small on paper (from 1 to 0.5, or from 0.5 to 0.25) turns out to be one of the hardest of the whole taper.

Common paroxetine withdrawal symptoms include severe brain zaps, marked dizziness, gait instability, gastrointestinal upset, sleep disturbance, and mood volatility. Anticholinergic rebound (increased sweating, altered bowel function, blurred vision) can also occur and is not always immediately recognised as withdrawal-related.

If your paroxetine taper produces severe symptoms that do not settle even with slow reductions, a fluoxetine bridge is worth discussing with your prescriber. This is one of the drugs where the bridge is most commonly used.

Two rules that apply across all the SSRIs

The first rule is that any reduction that produces symptoms severe enough to affect your daily functioning is a signal to hold, not to push through. Waiting at your current dose until the symptoms have fully settled is not a delay in your taper. It is your taper.

The second rule is that the schedules in this chapter are starting points, not sentences. If your body is telling you that the pattern is too fast, slow it down. If your body is telling you that it can absorb a larger cut, do not automatically take one; check with your prescriber, and if you both agree, adjust the schedule together.

Chapter 12 will give you the decision rules for when to hold, when to slow, and when to reinstate. Chapter 10 will give you a full symptom map so that when something new happens you know whether it is expected, unusual, or urgent.

The Named Principle of this chapter: the drug you are on has its own hyperbolic curve. Match your reductions to that curve, not to a rule of thumb that pretends every drug behaves the same.

In the next chapter, we look at the three SNRIs in this book, which behave differently enough from the SSRIs to need their own treatment.

Chapter 8: Coming Off SNRIs

The three SNRIs in this chapter (venlafaxine, duloxetine, and desvenlafaxine) share a family resemblance and one common problem. Their half-lives are, on the whole, shorter than those of the SSRIs. Venlafaxine's is about five hours. Duloxetine's is about twelve hours. Desvenlafaxine's is about eleven hours. Compared with fluoxetine's one-to-two-week metabolite half-life, these are all effectively short-half-life drugs.

Short half-life plus dual receptor action produces the characteristic SNRI withdrawal profile: rapid onset after missed or reduced doses, intensity that some patients describe as unlike anything else they have experienced, and a schedule of tapering that often has to be substantially slower than the SSRI schedules in Chapter 7.

If you are on one of these drugs and you are approaching your taper with some fear, that fear is not irrational. It is also not a reason to avoid the taper. It is a reason to plan it properly.

Venlafaxine (Effexor)

Venlafaxine is, by consensus, the most difficult common antidepressant in this book to come off. It combines the short half-life mentioned above with two other awkward features. Its active metabolite, O-desmethylvenlafaxine (also sold as desvenlafaxine), has slightly different pharmacokinetics. And the drug produces a well-documented and sometimes severe pattern of brain zaps and dizziness that begin within hours of a missed dose.

Standard tablet and capsule strengths of venlafaxine in most markets are 37.5, 75, and 150 mg. Some countries have 25 mg strengths. Below 37.5 mg, most patients need either a compounded liquid, bead counting from the extended-release capsules, or a fluoxetine bridge.

An example hyperbolic schedule from 75 mg:

Step	Dose (mg)	Time at Dose (weeks, minimum)
Starting	75	4
1	67	4
2	60	4
3	52	4
4	45	4
5	37.5	4
6	32	4
7	27	4
8	22	4
9	18	4
10	14	4
11	11	4
12	8	4
13	6	4
14	4	4
15	2.5	4
16	1.5	4
17	0.75	4
18	0	(final)

That is a long schedule, and it reflects the reality that venlafaxine tapers commonly take twelve to twenty-four months when done at a pace the nervous system can follow. If you have been on venlafaxine for many years or at a higher starting dose (150 mg or above), plan for the longer end of that range.

Bead counting is a common method for the middle and lower parts of a venlafaxine taper. A 75 mg extended-release capsule typically contains around 300 beads (this varies by manufacturer, and you should count your own capsule to check). Each bead is worth roughly 0.25 mg. A 10% reduction from 75 to 67 mg would mean removing roughly 30 beads. From 37.5 mg (typically around 150 beads), a 10% reduction to 33.75 mg would mean removing roughly 15.

Compounded liquid is the other common route, particularly for the bottom half of the taper. A liquid at 5 mg per ml lets you measure any dose from 0.5 mg upward with reasonable precision using a 1 ml syringe.

Common venlafaxine withdrawal symptoms include intense brain zaps (often triggered by eye movement), severe dizziness, gait instability, sweating, nausea, and marked emotional volatility. Sleep is often disturbed. Missed doses can produce full-onset withdrawal within twelve hours, which is a useful diagnostic test if you are ever uncertain about whether what you are feeling is drug-related: a rapid response to reinstatement (within hours) is highly suggestive.

If your venlafaxine taper produces symptoms that do not settle even with slow reductions, a fluoxetine bridge is a well-established option. The approximate cross-over involves stopping the venlafaxine, waiting a short period (typically a few days), and then starting fluoxetine at a dose your prescriber will work out. The fluoxetine is then tapered using the schedule in Chapter 7.

Duloxetine (Cymbalta)

Duloxetine sits close to venlafaxine in terms of tapering difficulty, though for most patients it is somewhat less severe. Its half-life is around twelve hours, which is longer than venlafaxine's but still short compared to the SSRIs.

Standard capsule strengths of duloxetine in most markets are 20, 30, and 60 mg. There is no widely available licensed liquid form in most countries. Bead counting is therefore the most common method for reaching doses below the smallest capsule.

Duloxetine capsules contain enteric-coated pellets that are designed to survive the stomach and dissolve in the small intestine. This is important: if you count beads, you must not crush or dissolve them, and you must swallow them intact. Some patients place the counted pellets into empty capsules for consistency.

An example hyperbolic schedule from 60 mg:

Step	Dose (mg)	Time at Dose (weeks, minimum)
Starting	60	4
1	54	4
2	48	4
3	42	4
4	36	4
5	30	4
6	25	4
7	20	4
8	16	4
9	12	4
10	9	4
11	6	4
12	4	4
13	2	4

Step	Dose (mg)	Time at Dose (weeks, minimum)
14	1	4
15	0	(final)

For higher starting doses (90 mg or 120 mg), the initial steps are proportionally larger. For the bottom of the taper, you may need a compounded formulation, or you may find, as some patients do, that the last small dose can be held for a longer stretch and then simply dropped.

Common duloxetine withdrawal symptoms overlap substantially with venlafaxine's: brain zaps, dizziness, nausea, sweating, mood volatility. Some patients report a distinctive pattern of vivid dreams and disrupted sleep that is more marked than with venlafaxine.

Desvenlafaxine (Pristiq)

Desvenlafaxine is the active metabolite of venlafaxine, sold as an antidepressant in its own right in some markets. It has a half-life of around eleven hours and is available primarily in 25, 50, and 100 mg tablet strengths.

The tablets are extended-release, and this creates a specific problem: they cannot be split, and there is no widely available licensed liquid form. This makes desvenlafaxine one of the more difficult drugs to taper below the smallest tablet strength, because none of the standard methods (splitting, bead counting, water titration) works cleanly.

The common solutions are compounded liquid (which requires a prescriber and a compounding pharmacy) or a switch to venlafaxine (which is the pro-drug that becomes desvenlafaxine in the body, and which comes in more flexible formulations).

An example hyperbolic schedule from 50 mg, assuming access to compounded liquid or a switch to venlafaxine:

Step	Dose (mg)	Time at Dose (weeks, minimum)
Starting	50	4
1	45	4
2	40	4
3	35	4
4	30	4
5	25	4
6	20	4
7	15	4
8	12	4
9	9	4
10	6	4
11	4	4
12	2	4
13	1	4
14	0	(final)

If you do not have access to compounded liquid, and if a switch to venlafaxine is not clinically appropriate, your prescriber may recommend a fluoxetine bridge as an alternative. This is a conversation to have specifically, because desvenlafaxine is one of the drugs where the formulation problem is most likely to shape the plan.

Common desvenlafaxine withdrawal symptoms are broadly similar to those of venlafaxine, though for many patients they are marginally less severe.

What all three SNRIs share

Three principles apply across all three SNRIs and are worth holding as a group.

First, missed doses are unusually consequential. Because the half-life is short and the withdrawal onset is rapid, forgetting to take an SNRI is not neutral. Set an alarm. Take it at the same time every day. If you do miss a dose, take it as soon as you remember, unless it is close to your next dose (in which case do not double-dose, but skip and continue as normal). Multiple missed doses in a row will produce full withdrawal, which is neither helpful nor safe.

Second, the first sign of a too-fast reduction is often gait instability or brain zaps rather than mood change. Watch for these physical signs early. They usually precede the mood volatility.

Third, formulation is more of a constraint with these drugs than with any others in this book. If you cannot get a workable formulation strategy in place before you start, you will not be able to complete the taper as planned. Solve the formulation question first; the schedule follows.

> **Important Point:** *If your prescriber does not know how to prescribe venlafaxine liquid, or does not know that bead counting is a recognised method, do not take that as the answer. Bring the evidence gently, request a referral to a psychiatrist familiar with deprescribing, or ask about a compounding pharmacy directly. This is a knowledge gap, not a policy.*

Hemi's venlafaxine schedule

Hemi had been on 150 mg of venlafaxine XR for six years, prescribed originally for panic disorder that had substantially resolved. He came in wanting to try coming off. He had heard, correctly, that venlafaxine was hard.

We planned his taper together over three appointments. He worked with his GP to switch from the once-daily 150 mg capsule to two 75 mg capsules, which gave him more flexibility for bead counting. His first reduction was from 150 to 135 mg, using bead counting from one of the two capsules. He held for four weeks. When he was ready, he reduced to 120 mg. He held again. He continued in this pattern, using the example schedule as a guide but slowing the intervals when symptoms lingered, until he reached 37.5 mg. At that point he switched to a compounded liquid at 5 mg per ml and completed the taper from there.

His total taper was nineteen months. He had two significant holds: one at 60 mg, when a family crisis made him unable to take on additional stress, and one at 4 mg, when a reduction to 2.5 mg produced a level of brain zaps he could not manage at work. He held at 4 mg for eight weeks, dropped to 3 mg for four weeks, and then continued to zero.

He said, at the end, "It was much harder than the SSRIs I had come off before. It was also not as bad as I had feared, mostly because we did not push through the difficult patches. When it was bad, we waited. When we made the cut, we knew the previous one had settled."

That principle, applied consistently over nineteen months, is what got him to zero.

The Key Takeaway of this chapter: SNRIs punish speed. Match the schedule to what the drug will absorb, and do not stack cuts on top of unsettled symptoms.

In the next chapter, we look at the two atypical antidepressants in this book (mirtazapine and trazodone) and the specific problem they both pose around sleep.

Chapter 9: Coming Off Mirtazapine and Trazodone

Mirtazapine and trazodone are grouped together in this chapter for one reason. In everyday clinical practice, both are prescribed most often at low doses for sleep, and both produce, when tapered, a specific pattern of rebound insomnia that dominates the withdrawal picture. Everything else in the withdrawal profile of these two drugs is secondary to that.

If you are on mirtazapine or trazodone at a higher dose for depression rather than at a low dose for sleep, the general principles below still apply, but you will encounter a slightly different symptom pattern. The core problem, however, remains: your sleep will change when you reduce, and if you do not plan for that, the taper will stall.

Mirtazapine (Remeron)

Mirtazapine acts on alpha-2 adrenergic autoreceptors, on serotonin receptors of several subtypes, and, importantly for sleep, on histamine H1 receptors. That last action is what makes it so sedating at low doses. At higher doses (30 or 45 mg), the noradrenergic and serotonergic effects become more prominent and, for many patients, mirtazapine actually becomes less sedating rather than more.

This has a specific implication for tapering. Reducing from 45 mg to 30 mg does not usually make you sleepier. Reducing from 15 mg to 7.5 mg often does, because at these lower doses the histamine-blocking sedation is proportionally larger. Reducing from 7.5 mg to zero often produces the biggest sleep disruption of the whole taper.

The half-life of mirtazapine is 20 to 40 hours, moderately long. Common tablet strengths are 15, 30, and 45 mg. An oro-dispersible form exists at similar strengths. Liquid formulations are available in some countries but not universally.

An example schedule from 30 mg:

Step	Dose (mg)	Time at Dose (weeks, minimum)
Starting	30	4
1	22.5	4
2	15	4
3	11	4
4	7.5	4
5	5.5	4
6	3.75	4
7	2.5	4
8	1.5	4
9	0.75	4
10	0	(final)

If you are on mirtazapine at 15 mg for sleep, you effectively start at step 2 of this schedule. If you are at 45 mg for depression, add an initial step at 37 mg before joining the schedule.

The rebound insomnia issue is worth thinking through in advance. In the weeks after a mirtazapine reduction, particularly at doses below 15 mg, you may find that falling asleep is harder, that you wake in the night, and that you have very vivid or unpleasant dreams. This is not the return of your original insomnia. It is the histamine system readjusting to the reduction in receptor blockade. It is real, and it is usually time-limited, but it can be disruptive.

Common mirtazapine withdrawal symptoms, in addition to sleep changes, include heightened anxiety (particularly in the first few days after a cut), vivid dreams, nausea, mild dizziness, and, in some patients, a return of appetite and food cravings after a period of reduced appetite. Bear in mind that some of these symptoms are the reverse of the drug's original effect: mirtazapine tends to increase appetite and encourage weight gain, so on the way out it can produce the opposite pattern.

> **Important Point:** *If you are on mirtazapine primarily for sleep, plan the taper around the sleep pattern. Consider whether you also want to introduce non-drug sleep supports (consistent bedtimes, light exposure in the morning, reduced screen time before bed) during the taper, so that when the drug is fully out you have a system in place.*

Trazodone

Trazodone at antidepressant doses (150 to 300 mg) works via serotonin reuptake inhibition and serotonin receptor antagonism. At the low doses at which it is now most commonly prescribed (25 to 100 mg for sleep), the receptor antagonism is dominant and the effect is largely sedating, similar in some respects to mirtazapine.

Its half-life is around seven to eleven hours, which is shorter than mirtazapine's. This makes trazodone somewhat quicker in onset of withdrawal after a missed dose, but also somewhat quicker to leave the system entirely, meaning that trazodone withdrawal typically resolves faster than mirtazapine withdrawal.

Common tablet strengths are 50, 100, 150, and 300 mg. Some countries have 25 mg or 75 mg strengths. A liquid form is available in some markets. Tablet splitting is generally reliable for the immediate-release form.

An example schedule from 50 mg (the typical low dose for sleep):

Step	Dose (mg)	Time at Dose (weeks, minimum)
Starting	50	3
1	37.5	3
2	25	3
3	18.75	3
4	12.5	3
5	6.25	3
6	3	3
7	0	(final)

For higher starting doses (150 or 200 mg for depression), the schedule extends proportionally.

Common trazodone withdrawal symptoms are dominated, at low doses, by sleep changes: difficulty falling asleep, night wakings, and occasionally vivid dreams. Some patients also report headaches, mild dizziness, and irritability. The syndrome is typically shorter than mirtazapine's, though this varies by person and by dose.

The sleep problem, in more detail

Both mirtazapine and trazodone are, in effect, functioning as sleep medications for a large number of patients. When you taper them, you are not just tapering an antidepressant; you are tapering the thing that has been getting you to sleep every night, in some cases for years.

There is no way to make this problem go away entirely. Rebound insomnia is real and, for most patients, is the price of coming off. What you can do is plan around it, so that the sleep disruption is time-limited, tolerable, and does not derail the taper.

Three strategies help. First, do not attempt the taper during a period when sleep is already precarious. If you are working night shifts, or you have a newborn, or you are travelling across time zones, wait. Second, put non-drug sleep supports in place before you start the taper. A consistent bedtime and wake time, exposure to bright light in the morning, avoidance of screens for an hour before bed, and reduction of alcohol and caffeine will not solve rebound insomnia by themselves, but they will substantially soften it. Third, expect the first two weeks after each reduction to be the hardest sleep-wise, and plan your work and family calendar to absorb it. If you can arrange for a slightly lighter workload in those weeks, do.

Some patients ask whether it is appropriate to take another sleep aid during the taper. This is a question to work through carefully with your prescriber. Some sleep aids have their own dependence profile and can create new problems. Others may be genuinely useful for a limited period. This is not a decision to make from a book; it is a decision to make with a clinician who knows your history.

What to expect after the last dose

The pattern of mirtazapine and trazodone recovery has one specific feature worth naming. For both drugs, the sleep disturbance may persist for weeks after the last dose. This does not mean the taper failed. It means that the histamine and serotonin receptor systems that regulate sleep are still readjusting. Most patients find that sleep normalises over a few weeks to a few months. A minority take longer.

If your sleep does not recover in the way you expected, this is a conversation to have with your prescriber. It does not automatically mean you need to go back on the drug, and it does not automatically mean you have developed a chronic sleep condition. It may mean that other factors (stress, alcohol, caffeine, screen use, general anxiety about sleeping) are keeping the problem going, and that these are workable. It may mean that you would benefit from a course of cognitive behavioural therapy for insomnia, which is a well-established non-drug treatment for insomnia and works for most people who try it. It may occasionally mean that some form of pharmacological support is appropriate again.

You do not have to answer that question from the middle of the difficult week. You will have better data after two months.

Alaria's mirtazapine taper

Alaria had been on 15 mg of mirtazapine for four years, prescribed originally for insomnia in the wake of a bereavement. Her sleep was, by the time she came in, generally reasonable, and she wanted to see whether she could sleep without the drug. She was in a stable relationship, in stable work, with no other stressors.

We planned her taper carefully. She read Chapter 4 and confirmed her readiness. She read Chapter 6 and worked out that her preferred method would be to switch from 15 mg tablets to oro-dispersible tablets, which she could split more reliably. She read this chapter and understood that the second half of the taper, from 7.5 mg downward, was likely to be where sleep disruption would show up.

She started in September, so that the difficult stretch would fall in the darker months when her sleep patterns were more forgiving anyway. Her first reduction from 15 to 11 mg was uneventful. Her second reduction to 7.5 mg produced two nights of poor sleep and then settled. Her third reduction, to 5.5 mg, produced two weeks of disrupted sleep. She held. Her sleep re-stabilised over three more weeks. She continued.

The reduction from 5.5 to 3.75 mg was the hardest of the taper. She had a fortnight in which she was waking at three in the morning and not falling asleep again. She held for six weeks. Over that time, she introduced the sleep supports we had discussed (morning light, consistent wake time, no phone in the bedroom). Her sleep gradually improved. When she was ready, she dropped to 2.5 mg, then to 1.5, then to 0.75, then to zero.

Her total taper was fourteen months. Her sleep took another eight weeks after the final dose to fully settle. At the end of that period, she was sleeping better than she had in years.

She said, "The thing I did not expect was that the taper taught me how to sleep without needing anything. I did not know I could do that."

That is a common experience, and a good one to end this chapter on.

The Named Principle of this chapter: mirtazapine and trazodone tapers are sleep tapers as much as they are drug tapers. Plan the sleep piece, and the rest usually follows.

In the next chapter, we look at the full withdrawal symptom map, so that you know what to expect and what should prompt urgent attention.

Chapter 10: The Withdrawal Symptom Map

This chapter is a map, not a menu. Its purpose is not to make you afraid of everything that might happen. Its purpose is to make sure nothing that happens is a shock.

Most people going through a well-planned taper will experience a subset of the symptoms in this chapter, at manageable intensity, for time-limited periods. A minority will experience symptoms outside this list, or symptoms in this list at severities that need active management. A very small minority will experience the protracted syndrome discussed in Chapter 13. This chapter covers what most people can expect. Chapter 13 covers what happens when the map does not cover the territory.

A general orienting fact before we start. Withdrawal symptoms typically emerge in the days following a dose reduction, peak within one to two weeks, and settle over the following weeks. Symptoms that persist unchanged for many weeks are either a signal that your reduction was too large (and you should discuss holding or reinstating) or, occasionally, a signal that something else is going on that is not withdrawal at all. This chapter helps you tell the difference.

Physical symptoms

Dizziness is the single most commonly reported physical withdrawal symptom. It can range from a mild lightheadedness on standing to a more persistent sense of being off balance. It is often worse on turning the head quickly and improves when you are still. For most patients it lasts days to a few weeks per reduction.

Brain zaps are, for those who get them, one of the most distinctive experiences of withdrawal. They are brief, shock-like sensations, often described as a jolt of electricity in the head, sometimes accompanied by a buzzing sound. They typically last a fraction of a second. They are often triggered by moving the eyes to the side, by turning the head, or by tiredness. They are not dangerous. They are not seizures. They are extremely unpleasant. They are also, for most patients, one of the earlier symptoms to settle after a reduction has been absorbed.

Flu-like symptoms are common. This can include fatigue, muscle aches, mild headache, sweating, and a general feeling of being unwell. If you have children, the shortest version of this is: you feel as though you might be coming down with something, and then you do not come down with anything.

Gastrointestinal upset (nausea, diarrhoea, occasional vomiting) is common in the first few days after a reduction, particularly with SNRIs. Small, plain meals often help. It typically settles within the first week.

Sensory disturbances (altered taste, altered smell, tinnitus, visual disturbances) are less common but well-documented. Light and sound sensitivity are among the most frequent. If a sensory symptom is new and does not settle over several weeks, mention it to your prescriber; while it may still be withdrawal-related, it is worth confirming that nothing else is going on.

Gait instability is a physical symptom that some patients find more distressing than the others, because it can affect driving, work, and daily function. It is most common with SNRI withdrawal. If it is severe enough to affect your ability to drive safely, you should not drive, and you should discuss the reduction with your prescriber.

Sleep symptoms

Sleep is one of the systems most affected by antidepressant taper. The main patterns to expect are:

Difficulty falling asleep. Even readers who had no sleep problems before starting the drug may find that in the days after a reduction, sleep onset is harder than usual.

Night wakings. Waking in the small hours and finding it hard to return to sleep is a common pattern, particularly on mirtazapine and trazodone tapers, and also on SSRI tapers late in the schedule.

Vivid dreams. Many patients describe unusually intense, coloured, or unsettling dreams during the taper. These are typically transient and pass within days or weeks per reduction.

Early morning waking. Waking at 4 or 5 am and not being able to sleep again is common. This is often mistaken for the return of depression, since early morning waking is a classic depression pattern. In withdrawal, however, it typically resolves as the reduction is absorbed.

Sleep management strategies were covered in Chapter 9 for the mirtazapine and trazodone tapers specifically. The same strategies (consistent bedtime, consistent wake time, morning light, reduced screen time) apply to SSRI and SNRI tapers.

Emotional symptoms

Emotional symptoms are perhaps the most important category to describe accurately, because they are the most easily confused with relapse and the most likely to be misinterpreted by the reader or the prescriber.

Heightened anxiety is common. You may find your anxiety threshold has lowered, so that things that would not have troubled you a month ago now do. This is different from the return of an anxiety disorder. Withdrawal-related anxiety is typically diffuse, not tied to specific triggers, and tends to fluctuate with the taper (worse in the days after a reduction, better as the reduction is absorbed).

Tearfulness is common. You may find yourself crying at things that do not seem to warrant it, or crying without a specific trigger. Some patients describe this positively, as feelings returning after a long stretch of numbness. Others find it exhausting. Both experiences are valid.

Irritability is common. Small things may seem larger. Traffic that would not have bothered you now does. Voices that would not have grated now grate. If you live with other people, it can help to tell them in advance that this pattern may show up so that they do not take it personally.

Emotional volatility is common, particularly at the bottom of the taper. You may find your mood swinging more than you are used to, from higher highs to lower lows within short time frames. This is generally time-limited and improves as the nervous system re-stabilises.

Rage or intense anger is less common but well-documented. Some patients describe waves of rage that feel disproportionate to the situation. This is a symptom that warrants specific attention: it can be frightening, it can cause damage to relationships, and it responds to a slower taper. If you notice this pattern, discuss it with your prescriber and consider slowing or holding.

Withdrawal-related low mood is one of the most complicated symptoms because it is the one most easily misread as relapse. The distinguishing features are that it typically emerges within days of a reduction, tends to fluctuate with reductions rather than to develop steadily over weeks, and often responds to a small reinstatement within days. Chapter 11 will help you tell these apart.

Cognitive symptoms

Brain fog, in the general sense, is common during withdrawal. You may find your working memory less reliable than usual, your ability to hold a train of thought less consistent, and your word-finding a bit slower. Most people find this less severe than they feared and it typically improves as reductions are absorbed.

Concentration difficulties are common. Reading a long article, watching a film, or completing a complex task at work may feel harder than it did a month ago. For many patients, this is one of the more manageable withdrawal symptoms. For some, particularly those in cognitively demanding work, it can be one of the harder ones.

Depersonalisation and derealisation (feeling as if you are not quite present in your own body, or that the world around you is not quite real) are less common but well-documented, particularly with SNRI tapers. These can be alarming. They are generally time-limited and improve. If they persist or become severe, they warrant a specific conversation with your prescriber.

Memory blips are common. Forgetting why you came into a room, misplacing your keys, momentarily forgetting a familiar name. These are the everyday version of brain fog. They almost always resolve.

Symptoms that warrant urgent attention

Most withdrawal symptoms, unpleasant as they are, do not require emergency care. A small number do, and you should know what they are.

Any thoughts of self-harm or suicide that feel more than fleeting, and particularly any thoughts that begin to feel like plans, are a signal to stop and reach out. Do not wait to see whether they pass. Call your prescriber. Call an urgent mental health crisis line (988 in the US; Samaritans 116 123 or NHS 111 in the UK; local equivalents elsewhere). If you feel unsafe alone, tell someone. There is no threshold you need to cross before you are entitled to help.

Severe agitation, particularly agitation combined with insomnia over several nights, warrants prescriber contact. Agitation of this kind can escalate quickly and is one of the more difficult withdrawal states to be in alone.

Marked functional collapse (you cannot get out of bed, cannot eat, cannot manage basic self-care) is a signal that the reduction has been too much for your current state. This is not a moral failure. It is a signal to reach out and to discuss slowing or reinstating.

Symptoms that seem physically unusual (chest pain, difficulty breathing, seizure-like activity, severe neurological signs) require immediate medical assessment, not because they are typical of antidepressant withdrawal, but because they may indicate something else entirely and should not be dismissed as withdrawal until they have been checked.

If in doubt, reach out. Prescribers would rather see a patient too early than too late.

> **Important Point:** *The single most useful sentence you can say to a prescriber during a difficult withdrawal is: "I am not planning anything. I want to tell you what I am feeling so we can adjust the plan." This gives them the clinical picture they need, without them having to make an emergency assessment.*

A note on suicidal ideation during withdrawal

Antidepressant taper can, in some patients, be associated with an increase in suicidal thinking. This is documented and it is not a sign that you are broken. It is a signal that your nervous system is under significant stress and that the current plan may need to be adjusted.

If you notice this pattern, please treat it as important information. Reach out to your prescriber. Reach out to a trusted person. Reach out to a crisis line if you need to. Consider slowing the taper, holding at the current dose, or reinstating a previous dose. None of these decisions require you to abandon the taper. They require you to adjust it in a way that keeps you safe.

This book will not, at any point, provide details of methods of self-harm. If you need urgent support, please use one of the resources named in the introduction and repeated in the appendices. You do not have to be certain you are in crisis to be entitled to help. Reaching out early is what keeps a difficult stretch from becoming something worse.

Ozias' symptom log

Ozias kept a daily log across his twelve-month escitalopram taper. He rated sleep, mood, and physical symptoms out of five each day, and wrote one sentence about how the day had gone.

Two months in, he had a rough week. He looked back at his log and realised something. He had had a similar rough week four weeks earlier, one week after a dose reduction. That week had passed. The current rough week was one week after the next dose reduction.

He was not, as he had briefly feared, spiralling. He was following a pattern.

Knowing this changed what he did. Instead of catastrophising, he waited. He kept up his sleep supports. He did not push himself at work. He talked to his partner. Ten days later, the rough patch was over, exactly as it had been the previous month.

That is what the symptom log buys you. It converts a bad day from a signal that everything is failing into a data point in a pattern you can read.

The Named Principle of this chapter: withdrawal is a set of expected physiological events with characteristic patterns.

Knowing the patterns lets you treat a bad day as data rather than as a verdict.

In the next chapter, we look specifically at how to tell withdrawal from relapse, which is the most consequential judgement of any taper.

Chapter 11: Withdrawal or Relapse

Phaedon had done everything by the book. He had drafted a plan with his GP. He had reduced his sertraline slowly, from 100 mg down to 25 mg over ten months. He had used a licensed liquid for the last three months. He had reached 5 mg, held for two months, and finally dropped to zero six weeks before the appointment where he sat in front of me looking exhausted.

He had been well for the first three weeks after the final dose. In the fourth week, his sleep had begun to erode. In the fifth week, a familiar heaviness had returned to his mornings. In the sixth week, he had woken up at 5 am with his chest tight and thought, quite clearly, that he could not do another day of this. He had come in wanting to know one thing: is this withdrawal, or is my depression coming back?

This question is the single most consequential judgement of a taper, and it is also the one that prescribers get wrong most often. Get it right, and you have a clear next step. Get it wrong, and you may either reinstate a medication you no longer need, or refuse to reinstate a medication that would prevent a serious relapse.

This chapter will give you a framework for making that judgement. It will not always give you a definitive answer, because the honest reality is that sometimes the picture is genuinely mixed. But it will give you the four dimensions to consider, a decision aid you can bring to your prescriber, and enough language to make the conversation productive.

The four dimensions

Withdrawal and relapse differ along four dimensions: timing, symptom pattern, response to reinstatement, and comparison with baseline. No single dimension is definitive on its own. Considered together, they usually produce a clear picture.

Timing. Withdrawal characteristically emerges within days of a dose change, most often within the first two weeks. Relapse characteristically emerges over weeks to months after a stable state has been reached, and its emergence is gradual rather than acute. If you cut your dose on Tuesday and by Friday you feel unwell, that is not the depression coming back. Depression does not develop over four days. If you finished your taper six weeks ago and your mood has been gradually declining, that pattern is more consistent with relapse.

Symptom pattern. Withdrawal characteristically includes physical and sensory symptoms that were not part of the original condition. Brain zaps. Dizziness. Nausea. Gait instability. Sensory changes. If your symptoms include these, that is a signal you are in withdrawal territory. Relapse characteristically resembles the original condition rather than a new symptom cluster. If your symptoms look like the depression or anxiety you had before you started the drug, and if they do not include the distinctive physical and sensory features, that is a signal you may be in relapse territory.

Response to reinstatement. Withdrawal characteristically responds to a small reinstatement of the drug within days. If reinstating a small dose produces noticeable improvement within a week, that is strong evidence of withdrawal. Relapse characteristically does not respond that quickly. It typically takes a therapeutic dose, taken for weeks, to produce clear improvement in a genuine relapse. This dimension is the most diagnostic of the four, though it requires you to actually make the reinstatement trial to test it.

Comparison with baseline. Ask yourself: does what I am feeling now look like what I felt before I started the drug in the first place, or does it look like something else? Many patients started their antidepressant for a specific reason (depression, panic, social anxiety, obsessive thoughts, post-traumatic stress). If what you are feeling now closely resembles what you were feeling then, that is a signal for possible relapse. If it does not resemble it, and particularly if the symptoms are unfamiliar or physical, that is a signal for withdrawal.

Working through the four dimensions with Phaedon

Phaedon and I went through the four dimensions together.

Timing. He had been well for three weeks after his final dose. The symptoms had emerged in the fourth to sixth weeks. That timing is atypical for acute withdrawal (which usually appears within two weeks) but is compatible with either late-emerging withdrawal (which can occur, particularly after long tapers) or early relapse (which can also emerge in the first two months). This dimension was ambiguous.

Symptom pattern. His symptoms were: early morning waking, low mood in the mornings, chest tightness, and a heaviness he described as "the exact feeling I had before I started the drug". No brain zaps. No dizziness. No sensory changes. This dimension pointed toward relapse.

Response to reinstatement. We had not tested this yet.

Comparison with baseline. Phaedon had originally started sertraline for what looked like a moderate depressive episode following the end of a long relationship. What he was describing now, he said, "felt more like that episode than anything else has in the last decade".

Three of the four dimensions pointed toward relapse. The fourth (response to reinstatement) we had not tested. I told him that in my judgement the picture was more consistent with an emerging depressive episode than with late withdrawal, and that we had two reasonable options. One was to reinstate sertraline at a low dose (something like 25 mg) and see whether the improvement was fast (favouring withdrawal) or slow and needing dose adjustment (favouring relapse). The other was to try a course of therapy first, monitor closely, and reinstate only if things worsened over the next several weeks.

Phaedon chose to reinstate at 25 mg. He improved over the next three weeks, then plateaued, then improved slightly again when we increased to 50 mg. That pattern, with its slow tempo, was more consistent with relapse than with withdrawal (which would have improved more rapidly on reinstatement).

He stayed on 50 mg. He is doing well. When we discussed it a year later, he was clear that reinstating had been the right call, and that he did not regret the taper attempt. He had learned that his depression was still there, and he had learned that a lower dose than his original 100 mg was enough. Both were useful pieces of information.

When the picture is genuinely mixed

Sometimes the four dimensions do not line up cleanly. Timing is compatible with either. Symptoms include some physical features but also some that resemble the original condition. There is no clear baseline to compare with because the original condition was diffuse. In these cases, the most useful move is often to conduct a small reinstatement trial and see what happens.

A reinstatement trial works like this. You go back to a dose you were on and stable at, or a moderate dose your prescriber suggests. You hold that dose for two to three weeks. If your symptoms improve substantially within days to a week, the case for withdrawal is strong. If they do not improve, or if they improve slowly and only over weeks, the case for relapse is stronger.

The reinstatement trial has one important caveat. If you reinstate at a dose lower than the one that produced withdrawal, and if you were far into the taper, sometimes even the correct diagnosis of withdrawal will produce only partial improvement, because the reinstated dose is too small. Discuss with your prescriber what dose to use for the trial. If they suggest a dose higher than the last one that felt stable, ask why.

The decision aid, in a single paragraph

If the symptoms began within two weeks of a dose change, include unusual physical or sensory features, and respond quickly to a small reinstatement, this is almost certainly withdrawal. If the symptoms emerged gradually over weeks after a stable state was reached, resemble the original condition rather than a new symptom cluster, and do not respond quickly to a small reinstatement, this is more likely to be relapse. If the picture is mixed, a small reinstatement trial is often the most useful next step. Regardless of which it turns out to be, you have not failed. You have simply learned what your nervous system needs.

Why prescribers get this wrong

For most of the past thirty years, medical training has not equipped prescribers to make this distinction reliably. The default assumption has often been that any symptom emerging after a dose reduction was either mild transient discontinuation (which would pass on its own) or relapse (which needed the drug to be restarted). The possibility of significant withdrawal, particularly withdrawal that could look like the original condition, was underappreciated.

The situation is improving. The 2019 Horowitz and Taylor paper in The Lancet Psychiatry, the wider dissemination of hyperbolic tapering, the 2024 deprescribing guidance published in the UK, and the growing patient advocacy movement have all contributed to a more nuanced view among clinicians who have kept up with the literature.

But not every prescriber has kept up. If you find yourself in front of a prescriber who is confidently telling you that what you are experiencing is relapse, and you are not sure they have considered the withdrawal possibility, it is reasonable to ask. You do not need to make an accusation. You can simply say, "I hear you saying you think this is relapse. Could we also talk about whether it might be withdrawal, and how we would tell?" That question, gently asked, tends to open a productive conversation.

Chapter 14 will give you a fuller script.

What if it turns out to be relapse

If, after working through the four dimensions and possibly conducting a reinstatement trial, the picture is genuinely one of relapse, this is not a failure of the taper. It is a piece of clinical information you did not have before. You may decide, together with your prescriber, that going back on the drug is the right move for now. You may decide to try a different medication, or add non-drug supports, or begin therapy, or all three.

Relapse is not shameful. Some proportion of patients who come off any medication for a chronic condition will experience recurrence, and this is not a moral event. It is a biological one. What matters is that you and your prescriber have made the decision with clear eyes, not on the basis of a misidentified withdrawal.

Some patients, having relapsed and restarted, decide never to attempt to come off again. That is a legitimate choice. Others decide to try again in a few years, using what they learned this time. That is also legitimate. There is no correct answer here. There is only your best judgement, made with your prescriber, on the basis of the picture in front of you.

What if it turns out to be withdrawal

If the picture is one of withdrawal, and if you are still committed to coming off, your next step is to make a decision between three options: hold at your current dose, slow the pace of future reductions, or reinstate a previous dose and start again more gently.

Chapter 12 will walk you through this decision in detail.

The Named Principle of this chapter: withdrawal and relapse are not the same thing, and the distinction lives in the pattern, the timing, and the response to reinstatement. Working through those three carefully will get you to the right answer more often than a snap judgement will.

In the next chapter, we look at how to actually make the hold, slow, or reinstate decision.

Chapter 12: When to Hold, When to Slow, When to Reinstate

Every taper will produce, at some point, a reduction that does not settle in the expected timeframe. This is not a failure of your plan; it is the plan meeting your specific nervous system on a specific week. What happens next is one of the most important choices you will make during the whole taper, and it comes in three forms: hold, slow, or reinstate.

Getting this choice right is not a matter of talent. It is a matter of following a small set of decision rules that convert the messy question of "am I okay?" into a more useful question of "what should I do next?"

The three options, in plain terms

Hold means staying at your current dose without further reductions until your symptoms have settled. It is the default option for most difficulties. A hold might last two weeks or three months. It ends when you have been symptom-free for at least a week or two and feel steady enough to consider the next cut.

Slow means, at the point of the next reduction, taking a smaller step than the plan called for. If the plan called for a 10% cut and you have just been through a difficult stretch, you might drop to a 5% cut for the next reduction, or reduce the size of subsequent cuts for the rest of the taper. Slowing is often paired with a hold: you hold first until symptoms settle, then slow the next step.

Reinstate means going back to a previous dose that you were stable at, or partway back to it, and holding there until you have re-stabilised before continuing. Reinstatement is the appropriate choice when a reduction has produced symptoms that are not settling with a hold at the new dose, or when the symptoms are severe enough that they need to resolve quickly rather than over an extended hold.

The decision rules

Rule one. If the symptoms from the last reduction are still present but appear to be improving over successive weeks, hold at the current dose. Time is doing what time does. You do not need to change thc plan; you need to wait.

Rule two. If the symptoms from the last reduction have been present for more than four to six weeks at the same intensity, without clear improvement, the reduction was too large. You have two options. You can hold at the current dose for a longer stretch (some patients continue to improve into the second month), or you can reinstate to a previous dose. Which you choose depends on how you are functioning at the current dose. If you can manage your daily life at the current dose while you wait, hold longer. If you cannot, reinstate.

Rule three. If, at any point during the taper, symptoms are severe enough that you cannot function (cannot work, cannot sleep, cannot manage self-care) and are not improving day by day, reinstatement is usually the right choice. You do not have to be in crisis to reinstate. Reinstatement is a tool, not a defeat.

Rule four. If you have thoughts of self-harm or suicide that feel more than fleeting, reinstate. Do not wait to see. Contact your prescriber and reinstate to a stable dose. Chapter 10 covered this specifically. The rule bears repeating here because this is the chapter where decisions are made.

Rule five. Once you have held or reinstated for long enough to be stable, when you resume the taper, make the next cut smaller than the one that produced the trouble. If a 10% cut destabilised you, try 5%. If 5% still produces symptoms, try 2.5%. This is not a sign of weakness. It is what a nervous system that is more sensitive than average is asking you to do.

How to reinstate, in practice

Reinstatement works best when it is done relatively soon after the destabilising reduction. The general observation is that reinstatement within a few weeks of the reduction produces reliable relief. Reinstatement done months later is less predictable: sometimes it works, sometimes the nervous system has moved on in ways that do not respond as expected. If you are considering reinstatement, do not delay to see what happens; delay is not neutral.

The dose you reinstate to is typically the last dose at which you were stable, or a dose partway between that and your current one. If you dropped from 20 mg to 15 mg and became unstable, reinstating to 20 mg (the last stable dose) is the standard move. Reinstating to 17.5 mg (partway) is an option if your prescriber prefers a smaller reinstatement, but the rule of thumb is that a small reinstatement often does not restore stability and you end up going up further anyway.

Once reinstated, hold at that dose for at least two to four weeks, and until you have been fully stable for at least a week or two. Then, if you still want to continue the taper, plan the next reduction more gently than the one that produced the destabilisation.

Reinstatement is not the end of the taper. Many patients reinstate one or two times during a long taper and still reach zero. It is a course correction, not a verdict.

When to hold, more specifically

Holding is the appropriate response to most manageable withdrawal patterns. It is the option that says: "my body is telling me it needs more time at this dose. I will give it more time."

Hold at the current dose when:

Symptoms from the last reduction are present but manageable, and you are still functioning in your daily life.

Symptoms are showing week-on-week improvement, even if slowly.

You are not in a life stretch that will exceed your capacity to wait.

You do not have thoughts of self-harm and are not experiencing severe agitation.

Holds typically last three to eight weeks. If a hold extends beyond eight weeks without meaningful improvement, that is your signal that reinstatement, not further waiting, is likely the right move.

Holds are also the correct response to external life events during a taper. If a family crisis, a work crisis, or a major transition arrives partway through the taper, holding at your current dose until the crisis has passed is generally wise, even if you were about to make the next reduction. The taper can wait; life often cannot.

When to slow, more specifically

Slowing is the response to a taper that is generally working but is producing more turbulence than you want. You have been getting through, but the reductions are hitting harder than expected, and you would like the ride to be smoother.

Slow the pace of future reductions when:

You have completed several reductions and are consistently having a rougher time than you expected.

You are approaching the bottom of the taper, where the receptor curve is at its steepest.

Your life circumstances are demanding more from you than they were at the start of the taper.

Slowing does not mean making the whole taper slower in principle. It means making the next few cuts smaller and, if needed, longer between cuts. The plan is adjusted; the taper continues.

What to do at the appointment

If you have decided that a hold, slow, or reinstatement is appropriate, the appointment with your prescriber has three parts.

First, describe what you are experiencing in plain language. Not "I think I need to reinstate" but "For the last three weeks I have had brain zaps every day, my sleep has collapsed, and I cannot concentrate at work. This started ten days after I reduced from 15 to 10 mg." Facts, dates, patterns.

Second, name your interpretation. "I think this is too large a reduction for me at this stage. I would like to reinstate to 15 mg, hold until stable, and then plan smaller cuts from there."

Third, ask for their view. "Does that make sense to you? Is there something else I should be considering?"

If they agree, you write the new plan together. If they suggest something different, listen. They may know something you do not. They may also be reaching for the older tapering advice by habit, in which case Chapter 14 has scripts for gently redirecting. Either way, the conversation is a negotiation, not a submission.

> **Important Point:** *Do not present the decision as "I have failed." Present it as "The plan needs adjustment based on what my body is telling us." One framing invites reassurance; the other invites collaboration.*

The trap of pushing through

There is a specific trap worth naming. Some patients, having got this far, become invested in completing the taper on the timeline they originally set. They may resist holding when a hold is appropriate. They may resist reinstating because it feels like going backward. They may push through symptoms that a slower approach would resolve.

Pushing through does not, in most cases, produce a faster taper. It produces a taper with more destabilisation, more damage to daily life, and a higher probability of eventually needing a longer reinstatement or of losing the whole attempt.

The taper is not something you win. It is something you navigate. The person who reaches zero six months later than they planned, having held twice, has done a better taper than the person who reaches zero on time by pushing through and ends up on a higher dose than they started at six months after that.

Give yourself permission to slow down.

What if reinstatement does not work

For a small minority of patients, reinstatement does not produce the expected recovery. The dose that was previously stable no longer feels stable, or the improvement is partial, or new symptoms emerge that were not there before.

This is uncommon, and it is difficult when it happens. If you find yourself in this position, the immediate priorities are safety and support. Work closely with your prescriber. Consider referral to a specialist familiar with deprescribing if one is available. Consider whether other supports (therapy, sleep management, temporary help with daily life) are needed while things stabilise.

Chapter 13 covers protracted withdrawal, which is the situation for some patients where symptoms persist over months to years. If you find yourself heading in that direction, that chapter is where to go next.

Most reinstatements work. If yours does not, you are not alone, and you are not without options.

Bindi's second appointment

Bindi, whom you met in Chapter 1 with her citalopram, hit a difficult stretch six months into her taper. She had been reducing steadily, then dropped from 8 mg to 6 mg and was miserable for three weeks. She came back in and said, "I think I need to hold. I don't want to reinstate, but I can't do the next cut yet."

We looked at her log. She was functioning, if barely. Her mood was low but not dangerous. Her sleep was disturbed but not collapsed. She had been improving, week by week, but slowly.

I agreed with her assessment. She held at 6 mg for eight weeks. She continued to improve. When she was ready, she dropped to 5.25 mg instead of the 5 mg the plan had called for. That smaller cut settled within two weeks. She continued in smaller steps for the rest of the taper.

Her whole taper took eighteen months instead of the twelve to fourteen we had originally sketched. She reached zero without needing to reinstate. She said, "That eight-week hold was the best decision I made during the whole thing. It made everything after it easier."

That is what holding buys you.

The principle of this chapter: hold, slow, or reinstate are not admissions of defeat. They are the tools that let a good taper stay a good taper when your nervous system says it has had enough for now.

In the next chapter, we look at protracted withdrawal, which is what happens when the map does not cover the territory.

Chapter 13: Protracted Withdrawal, An Honest Chapter

This chapter is different from the ones before it. Most of this book has described what usually happens when antidepressants are tapered carefully. This chapter is about what happens for the minority of patients for whom "usually" does not apply.

Protracted withdrawal is the term used in the current literature for a withdrawal syndrome that persists for months to years after the drug has been stopped. It is not common, and I will give you the numbers we have in a moment. It is also not, as it was once dismissed as being, a psychosomatic reaction or a return of the original condition. It is a documented phenomenon with a growing evidence base, and any book on antidepressant tapering that pretended it did not exist would be doing you a disservice.

I want to be careful about how I write this chapter, because the two errors I want to avoid are opposite. The first error would be to frighten you into abandoning a taper you would probably complete without significant trouble. The second would be to leave you without the information you need if you turn out to be one of the small number of patients for whom the picture becomes more complicated than the earlier chapters describe. I am going to try to walk the line between those two errors by telling you what is known, honestly.

What we mean by protracted withdrawal

A working definition, drawn from the recent literature: protracted withdrawal is a syndrome that emerges during or after tapering, involves symptoms consistent with the withdrawal profile of the drug (physical, sensory, sleep, emotional, cognitive), persists for more than several weeks after the last dose reduction or the last dose, and does not respond in the expected way to reinstatement.

Some authors use the term post-acute withdrawal syndrome, or PAWS, borrowed from the substance-use literature. Some use protracted antidepressant withdrawal syndrome, or PAWS in a different formulation. Others use post-SSRI withdrawal or post-discontinuation withdrawal. The literature has not yet fully settled on a single term. What matters is the underlying phenomenon: a small number of patients experience a withdrawal picture that outlasts the timeframes described in Chapter 10.

The picture is heterogeneous. Some patients experience persistent sensory disturbances (visual snow, tinnitus, altered smell). Some experience persistent cognitive changes (brain fog, memory difficulties, word-finding problems). Some experience persistent mood changes (dysthymia, anhedonia, emotional blunting or emotional volatility). Some experience persistent physical symptoms (fatigue, muscle pain, gastrointestinal issues, sexual dysfunction). Many experience combinations. What unifies these presentations is time: symptoms that would normally settle within weeks are still present at three months, six months, sometimes years.

What we know about how often this happens

The honest answer is that we do not have a definitive base rate. What we have is a set of imperfect estimates from several sources, and they do not fully agree.

The largest patient-reported dataset comes from the online peer communities that emerged during the 2010s as a place for patients whose experiences were not being recognised in mainstream care. The Surviving Antidepressants forum and its counterparts have collected many thousands of self-reported cases. These cases confirm that protracted withdrawal exists and give a rich picture of what it can look like, but as a source of prevalence data they are limited by the fact that people who are having a straightforward experience of tapering are less likely to seek out these communities. The population represented is skewed toward difficult experiences.

More systematic estimates come from a smaller number of clinical and academic studies. A survey analysis by Hengartner and colleagues, published in 2020, examined 69 people reporting protracted withdrawal and found that symptoms had persisted for between five and 166 months, with a median of 26 months. A more recent systematic review published in 2025 identified persistent post-withdrawal syndromes as a real but under-quantified phenomenon and called for better prospective research. Older estimates by Fava and colleagues suggested that some form of post-acute or protracted withdrawal might affect a meaningful minority of long-term users, though the precise proportion varies by study and by how the syndrome is defined.

The rate of protracted withdrawal is almost certainly higher in patients who tapered quickly and lower in patients who tapered slowly, but the relationship is not perfectly clean, and some patients experience protracted symptoms even after slow tapers. It also appears to be more common in long-term users (many years of exposure) than in short-term users.

If I had to give you a working figure, I would say that the risk of some form of protracted withdrawal in a slowly-tapered long-term user is probably in the low single-digit percentages, and possibly higher in populations with fast tapers or particular drugs. This is an estimate, not a fact, and I would rather give you an honest estimate than a false precision.

Who is at higher risk

The following factors are associated with a higher risk of protracted symptoms, based on the current literature.

Long duration of use. Users who have been on the drug for many years appear to be at higher risk than short-term users.

Fast tapering. Users who came off over weeks are at higher risk than users who came off over many months. Chapter 3's argument for hyperbolic tapering is, in part, an argument for reducing this risk.

Prior difficult tapers. Users who have had significant withdrawal on previous taper attempts appear to be at higher risk on subsequent attempts, though the mechanism is not fully understood.

Higher doses. Users who tapered from higher doses appear to be at somewhat higher risk than users who tapered from lower doses.

Specific drugs. Paroxetine and venlafaxine appear to be associated with higher rates of protracted symptoms, consistent with their status as the most difficult drugs in this book to come off.

Being on multiple psychiatric medications. Users tapering off an antidepressant while also on other psychiatric drugs (benzodiazepines, antipsychotics, mood stabilisers) appear to be at higher risk of complicated presentations.

Some of these risk factors are modifiable and some are not. If you have several, that is not a reason not to taper. It is a reason to taper more slowly, with more support, and with your prescriber as a genuine partner.

What protracted withdrawal can look like

I want to describe, briefly, the shape of what patients report, so that if you find yourself in this territory you will recognise it and know it has been described.

Sensory persistence. Some patients report that sensory changes (light sensitivity, sound sensitivity, altered taste or smell) do not settle in the weeks after the taper but continue for months. Visual snow, a specific phenomenon in which the visual field appears to have a persistent grainy quality, is reported by some patients.

Cognitive persistence. Some patients report that brain fog, difficulty concentrating, and word-finding problems continue at levels beyond what would be expected in acute withdrawal.

Emotional flatness or blunting. This is one of the most complicated of the persistent symptoms. Some patients describe an ongoing sense that their emotional range is reduced, that they do not feel joy or grief as they used to, and that this state persists long after the drug is gone. The literature on post-SSRI emotional blunting is developing.

Sleep changes. Persistent insomnia or unrefreshing sleep can continue for months in some patients.

Physical persistence. Fatigue, muscle pain, headaches, and gastrointestinal changes can persist. Some patients report a distinctive physical state that they describe as feeling constantly unwell without a specific illness.

Sexual dysfunction. A specific syndrome, post-SSRI sexual dysfunction, has been recognised in the literature as a potentially persistent condition for a small number of patients. It is documented as an ongoing area of research and clinical concern, and there is a growing body of work on it that is separate from the general withdrawal literature.

None of these patterns is universal. Most patients who experience protracted symptoms experience only a subset of these, and most eventually improve, though the timeframe can be long.

What tends to help

This is the honest section, because the honest answer is that we do not yet have a well-established treatment protocol for protracted withdrawal. What we have is a set of clinical observations and patient reports about approaches that have helped some people some of the time.

Time. This is the most consistent finding. The majority of protracted cases improve, though improvement can be measured in months to years rather than weeks. This is difficult to hear when you are in the middle of it. It is also, for most patients, what happens.

Nervous system regulation supports. Practices that support the parasympathetic nervous system (slow breathing, gentle exercise, regular sleep-wake times, minimal alcohol and caffeine, adequate protein and micronutrient intake) tend to be reported as helpful by patients who eventually improve. These are not cures. They are foundational supports that create the conditions in which recovery can occur.

Trauma-informed and body-based therapies. Approaches that work with the nervous system rather than only with cognition (somatic experiencing, sensorimotor psychotherapy, and related approaches) are reported by many patients as helpful for the physical and sensory aspects of protracted withdrawal. Evidence remains largely observational.

Careful reinstatement. In some cases, a small reinstatement at a low dose can improve symptoms enough to allow the patient to stabilise and taper again more slowly. This is not always successful, and the decision has to be made carefully with a prescriber familiar with the phenomenon.

Peer support. Many patients report that connection with others who have been through similar experiences is one of the most important sources of hope and practical guidance. Peer communities specifically for post-antidepressant withdrawal have been documented as significant sources of support, and they are named in the appendices.

Time again. It is worth saying twice. Many patients, looking back after two or three years, describe a slow but steady recovery. The trajectory is not linear (there are windows and waves, better days and worse) but the overall arc, for most, is upward.

> **Important Point:** *If you find yourself in protracted withdrawal, the first task is not to identify the intervention that will fix it. It is to stabilise your life around it (sleep, food, movement, connection) and give your nervous system the time and conditions it needs. Interventions can come later. The stabilising work is the ground on which anything else will stand.*

What does not usually help

For completeness, some things worth naming.

Chasing multiple new medications in an attempt to control the symptoms rarely helps and often adds complexity. Each new drug is a new variable with its own withdrawal profile.

Rapidly cycling reinstatements (starting a drug, stopping when it seems to help, restarting when symptoms return) tend to destabilise rather than stabilise. If a reinstatement is going to be tried, it should be planned and held.

Alcohol as a management strategy tends to produce worse symptoms overall, even if it seems to help in the immediate moment.

Isolation is one of the most reliable predictors of a worse subjective experience of protracted withdrawal. The pull to isolate is understandable and strong. Resisting it, in small ways, matters.

When to seek specialist support

If you find yourself with symptoms that persist beyond three to six months after your last dose or last reduction, and if those symptoms are affecting your daily life, it is time to seek specialist support if you have not already. The right specialist is a psychiatrist or GP with experience in deprescribing and withdrawal syndromes, and such clinicians are still not everywhere. If your regular prescriber is not that person, ask for a referral, or seek out a specialist clinic if one is available in your country.

The support you need may involve medical management, but it may also involve therapy that is trauma-informed and pace-sensitive, occupational adjustments to allow you to work at a reduced tempo, and connection with a peer community. A good specialist will help you think about all of these, not only the medical piece.

You are not too complicated to help. The picture may be difficult, but it is not outside the range of what specialists in this area have seen and worked with before.

A note on hope, honestly framed

Protracted withdrawal is difficult. I do not want to minimise it, and if you are reading this chapter because you are in it, I know that no reassurance from a book will substitute for what you are actually experiencing.

I also want to be truthful about what is known. Most patients who develop protracted symptoms eventually improve. Improvement is often slower than the patient wants, and there can be setbacks along the way, but the overall trajectory for most is upward. Some patients recover fully. Some recover partially and adapt. A small number continue to experience significant symptoms long-term.

The literature on long-term outcomes is still developing, and I will not pretend it is more definitive than it is. What I can tell you is that the picture is not hopeless, that the field is paying more attention to this problem than it did even five years ago, and that patient advocacy has driven substantial changes in the way withdrawal is now recognised and researched.

If you are in this territory, you are not alone, you are not imagining it, and you are not permanently broken. You are in a hard place, and that hard place is beginning to be understood.

The Important Point of this chapter: protracted withdrawal is real, uncommon but not rare, and best met with stability, time, and support rather than with panic or with the assumption that nothing can be done.

In the next chapter, we turn to the conversation with your prescriber, which is one of the most important pieces of infrastructure for both the routine and the difficult stretches of the whole taper.

Chapter 14: Talking to Your Prescriber

This is the practical chapter. By the time you have reached it, you have a plan, a formulation strategy, an understanding of the withdrawal profile, and a framework for the decisions that will come up along the way. What you may not yet have is the language to bring all of this into a ten-minute appointment with a prescriber whose training may have covered rather different assumptions.

This chapter gives you five scripted conversations, each written out in the words you can actually use. They are not scripts to memorise word for word. They are scripts to sit with, adapt to your voice, and take into the room. Their purpose is to convert the emotional weight of the request ("please take me seriously") into a clinical structure that a prescriber can respond to as a colleague rather than as a source of anxiety.

At the end of the chapter is a one-page evidence handout you can print or copy and take with you. It contains the key references that support the conversation and can be handed across the desk if useful.

Script one: asking for a slower taper than the leaflet recommends

The situation. You are on a moderate dose of an SSRI. Your prescriber has agreed you can try coming off. They have suggested a schedule of two dose reductions over four to six weeks. You have read this book and understand that this is much faster than the pharmacology of low-dose reduction supports.

The script.

"Thank you for supporting me in coming off. I have been reading about how the receptor occupancy changes at low doses, and I understand that reductions in milligrams at the bottom of the dose range produce much bigger changes in effect at the receptor than the same reductions at the top. Because of that, I would like to plan a slower taper than the leaflet describes, particularly at the lower doses.

"I have drafted a schedule I would like you to look at. It starts with 10% reductions of the current dose each month, and it gets to smaller reductions toward the end. The whole taper is planned to take about twelve months, longer if I need to hold at any point.

"How does that sound to you? Is there anything in my particular history that would make you want to adjust it?"

The reasoning behind the script. You have led with your understanding of the pharmacology, briefly and without lecturing. You have named the specific plan you want. You have invited their clinical judgement into the discussion. You have not challenged their competence. You have simply offered a more current framework and asked what they think of it.

Most prescribers, given this framing, will engage constructively. Some will want to adjust the plan. Some will want to see one of the sources you have read. The one-page handout at the end of this chapter is for those conversations.

Script two: asking for a switch to a liquid formulation

The situation. You are on a dose that will soon go below the smallest available tablet strength of your drug. You need to switch to a liquid to reach the smaller doses.

The script.

"I am going to be reducing below the smallest tablet strength soon. To do that accurately, I would like to switch to the liquid form of the drug. It is available at [concentration you have looked up]. The pharmacy [name if known] can order it in.

"Once I am on the liquid, I will measure my dose with the syringe that comes with it. That way I can reduce in the small steps my plan calls for without having to split tablets.

"Would you be willing to write the prescription for the liquid version?"

The reasoning. You have done the homework. You have named the specific formulation, checked availability, and identified the pharmacy. You have made it easy for the prescriber to say yes. If they hesitate, common reasons are unfamiliarity with the liquid, uncertainty about the concentration, or concern about cost. The unfamiliarity can be addressed by writing the specific product name and strength on a piece of paper for them. The concentration and dosing questions are addressed by the manufacturer's product information, which the pharmacy will confirm. Cost is a real issue in some healthcare systems and may need to be discussed frankly.

Script three: asking for a hold rather than pushing on

The situation. You reduced two weeks ago and are having significant symptoms that have not settled. Your prescriber has suggested continuing with the next reduction next month as planned. You believe you need to hold at the current dose until symptoms fully settle before making the next cut.

The script.

"I want to talk about what has been happening since the last reduction. I have had [name the symptoms: brain zaps, dizziness, sleep disturbance, mood changes, whatever your log shows] every day for the past two weeks. They are not yet settling.

"Based on that, I do not think I can move to the next reduction on schedule. I would like to hold at the current dose until the symptoms have been gone for at least a week, and only then plan the next step. That might mean waiting another four weeks. It might mean longer.

"Can we do that? And can we make the next reduction, when we get there, a bit smaller than the plan called for?"

The reasoning. You have described the symptoms concretely. You have named your interpretation and the change you would like to make. You have proposed both a specific action (hold) and a specific plan for the next step (smaller cut). This gives your prescriber a fully articulated proposal to respond to, rather than an anxious question that they might reflexively answer with reassurance and the original plan.

Script four: asking about reinstatement

The situation. You reduced several weeks ago, symptoms have been severe, and holding at the current dose has not led to improvement. You believe you should reinstate to your previous stable dose.

The script.

"I have held at the current dose for [number of weeks]. The symptoms have not settled. I am struggling to function at work and my sleep has not recovered. I do not think holding is working for me.

"I would like to reinstate to my previous dose of [X mg], which is where I was stable before this reduction. Once I am stable there, I would like to hold for a while longer than we originally planned, and then take smaller steps for the rest of the taper.

"Does that make sense to you? Would you write the prescription for the previous dose?"

The reasoning. Reinstatement is often the most sensitive conversation, because the patient may feel they are going backward, and the prescriber may reach for the older assumption that persistent symptoms after a reduction mean relapse. Naming the reinstatement as a course correction rather than a defeat, and naming the pattern that has led you to want it, gives the prescriber a clinical picture to work with.

If the prescriber wants to interpret the symptoms as relapse and start a different treatment, the framework from Chapter 11 (the four dimensions) is the response. You can say, "Before we treat this as relapse, could we look at the timing, the symptom pattern, and whether a small reinstatement would help? If it does, that would tell us something."

Script five: raising a concern about how withdrawal is being interpreted

The situation. Your prescriber, on hearing about your symptoms, has said that the depression is coming back and has suggested going back on the drug at a higher dose. You believe the picture is more consistent with withdrawal, based on Chapter 11.

The script.

"I hear you saying that this looks like the depression coming back, and I understand why you might think that. I would like to talk through whether it might also be withdrawal, because the treatment we choose depends on which it is.

"The symptoms started two days after I reduced my dose. They include [physical symptoms, sensory symptoms, whatever you have]. Those are not things I had when I was originally depressed. When I was depressed, I did not have brain zaps or dizziness. This feels physically different.

"Before we decide it is relapse, could we try a small reinstatement first, back to my last stable dose? If that improves things within a week, we would know it was withdrawal. If it does not, we would have information for the relapse question."

The reasoning. You have not contradicted the prescriber. You have taken their view seriously, offered an alternative interpretation, and proposed a diagnostic test (the reinstatement trial) that would produce information either way. This is exactly the kind of collaborative reasoning good clinicians appreciate. A clinician who resists this framing entirely is showing you something about their willingness to think about the problem, and you may want to consider whether they are the right prescriber for the rest of the taper.

The evidence handout, in one page

If, at any point in these conversations, your prescriber wants to see the evidence for hyperbolic tapering, receptor occupancy, or the recognition of protracted withdrawal, here is a compact summary you can print and hand over. It has been kept deliberately brief.

For hyperbolic tapering and the receptor occupancy science, the foundational paper is Horowitz and Taylor (2019) in The Lancet Psychiatry, titled "Tapering of SSRI treatment to mitigate withdrawal symptoms." The 2024 update by Horowitz and Taylor is the current clinical guidance most commonly cited internationally.

For the recognition of withdrawal as a physical dependence phenomenon distinct from addiction and from relapse, Fava and colleagues have published extensively since the 1990s, and their more recent reviews are the standard reference for the acute and post-acute presentations.

For the specific existence of protracted withdrawal, Hengartner and colleagues (2020) provides the most systematic published survey data available at the time of this book's writing, and the 2025 systematic review on post-acute withdrawal symptoms provides an updated synthesis.

For patient-reported perspectives that have shaped clinical understanding, the online peer community at Surviving Antidepressants provides thousands of documented case histories.

These references are also listed in the References section at the back of this book. Chapters 1 through 13 draw on these sources throughout.

What if your prescriber will not engage

If, having tried these conversations, your prescriber remains unwilling to support a slow taper, unwilling to consider withdrawal as a diagnosis, or unwilling to work with you on hold or reinstatement decisions, you have three options.

The first is to try again with a different framing, or after bringing evidence, or after a few weeks. Sometimes an initial reluctance softens with time and repeated conversation.

The second is to ask for a referral to a psychiatrist, or to a specialist deprescribing clinic if one is available in your country. In many healthcare systems, GPs can refer to specialists for exactly this kind of situation.

The third is to change prescribers. This is a real option, and while it is a significant step, it is preferable to attempting a taper without adequate medical support. If you are in a country where you can request a change of GP or find a psychiatrist directly, and if the current prescriber is not willing to work with you, changing is often the right move.

You may feel disloyal considering this, particularly if the prescriber has helped you in the past. Remember that you are asking for medical care that is aligned with current evidence, that this is a reasonable request, and that a prescriber who cannot or will not provide it is not the right prescriber for this stage of your treatment.

What a good taper conversation looks like

To end this chapter on the positive rather than the difficult, let me describe what a good conversation with a supportive prescriber can look like.

You come in with your log and your plan. You describe what has been happening since the last visit in specific terms. You name the decision you think needs to be made. Your prescriber listens, asks a question or two, offers their clinical view, and you agree together on the next step. The appointment takes fifteen minutes. You leave with a prescription that matches the plan, a follow-up date in the calendar, and the sense that the two of you are working the problem together.

That kind of appointment is possible, and it is increasingly common as the field shifts. If you are lucky enough to have a prescriber with whom you can have that kind of conversation, tell them, at some point during the taper, that you appreciate them. The kind of care they are giving is not the default, and they will appreciate knowing it makes a difference.

The Named Principle of this chapter: your prescriber is your most important taper partner, and the conversation with them is best served by clear language, concrete data, specific proposals, and mutual respect.

In the next chapter, we look at what it takes to keep the rest of your life running while you are doing all of this.

Chapter 15: Life During the Taper

The taper is not a project you do in a room by yourself. It happens during your ordinary life. Work continues. Children continue. Bills continue. Relationships continue. The house needs cleaning and the shopping needs doing. What the taper adds is a nervous system that is less reliably regulated than usual, and a set of decisions about how to protect the things that matter while your body works through its adjustment.

This chapter is about the practical mechanics of keeping the rest of your life running while you taper. It is not a self-improvement chapter. It is a chapter about triage: what to prioritise, what to let go, what to plan for, and what to say to the people around you.

Sleep, again

Sleep is the single most protective factor across a taper, and it is also one of the things withdrawal tends to disturb. This creates the specific difficulty that the times you most need sleep to be reliable are the times when it is least reliable.

The strategies from Chapter 9 apply here regardless of which drug you are on. Consistent bedtime and wake time. Morning light exposure. Reduced screen time in the hour before bed. Alcohol and caffeine kept moderate and away from evening hours. A dark, cool room. If you share a bed, an honest conversation about what you both need during the difficult stretches.

The temptation, during a bad sleep stretch, is to lie in bed trying to force sleep. This tends to make things worse. If you have been in bed for around 30 minutes and are not asleep, get up, do something quiet and undemanding in low light, and go back to bed when you feel drowsy. This is a cognitive behavioural therapy for insomnia technique and it works.

If sleep collapses for more than a week and is not improving, talk to your prescriber. Do not spiral. Do not decide at 4 am that the taper is failing. Look at your log; note the pattern; wait for a normal-hours conversation with someone who can help.

Work

Work during a taper is a matter of matching what you can absorb to what your work requires.

For jobs that permit some flexibility, the taper can be done during ordinary work. The main adjustments are pacing (do not schedule the most demanding projects for the two weeks after a reduction), transparency where trust allows (some people tell one colleague or their line manager that they are going through a medical adjustment; some do not), and self-protection (accept that some days will be quieter output than others, and do not try to make up for a slow day with a punishing next day).

For jobs that do not permit flexibility (frontline healthcare, high-stakes decision-making under time pressure, safety-critical roles), the calculation is different. Some patients in these roles schedule tapers around planned leave. Some reduce hours during the taper. Some, if the workload is unusually intense, wait until a career transition provides a natural window. The trap to avoid is proceeding under the assumption that you will simply be able to power through and finding out too late that you cannot.

If you are self-employed, or on a zero-hours or gig contract, the challenge is that your income depends on your capacity to work at a consistent level. This is worth planning for. Some patients build up a small financial buffer before starting a taper so that a slower two weeks is affordable. Some structure the taper so that the harder cuts fall in seasonally slower periods.

Driving is a specific point. Withdrawal-related dizziness or gait instability can affect driving safety. If you are having those symptoms, do not drive. Arrange for a lift, use public transport, or work from home if possible. This is not paranoia. It is what any sensible person does when their reaction time is not what it usually is.

Family and household

If you live with other people, especially a partner or children, the taper affects them too. They may notice that you are more irritable, more tired, more up and down. They may worry. They may take it personally when they should not.

The most useful conversation to have, before you start the taper or in its early weeks, is a conversation that tells them what is happening, why you are doing it, what to expect, and what you would like from them. This does not have to be a formal sit-down. It might be a walk, or a drive together, or an evening at home. What matters is that they hear it from you, in advance, rather than trying to work it out later from indirect signals.

For a partner, the conversation might sound something like: "I am coming off my antidepressant. I have a plan with my doctor. It is going to take about a year. There will be some patches where I am more irritable than usual, or sleeping less well, or feeling low. That is expected, and it is temporary. If I am short with you, it is not because I am angry with you; it is because the taper has taken a bad day. I would appreciate you not taking it personally, and I would appreciate you telling me if you notice I am struggling and not talking about it. If at any point you are seriously worried about how I am doing, please tell me, and I will take it seriously."

For children old enough to understand, an age-appropriate version might be: "Mummy is coming off a medicine she has taken for a long time. Sometimes she might be a bit tired or a bit grumpy, and that is because of the medicine changes, not because of anything you did. If you notice, you can tell me, and we can talk about it."

Children do not need clinical detail. They need honesty about the fact that something is changing, and reassurance that they are not the cause.

If you live alone, this conversation is worth having with one or two trusted friends, at least in general terms. You do not want to reach a difficult week with no one who knows to check in.

Emotional reappearance

One of the specific and less-discussed features of coming off long-term antidepressants is that emotional experiences you had not had for a long time may reappear. This can be a positive thing (a full-throated laugh, a wave of grief for someone you lost years ago, unexpected tears at a piece of music). It can also be disorienting, particularly if you had been on the drug for many years and had partially forgotten what your unmedicated emotional range felt like.

The reappearance of feeling is not, in general, a sign that anything is going wrong. It is often, in fact, one of the things patients most valued about coming off. But it can be surprising, and it can be intense. Give yourself space for it. Notice what is coming back. Some things you may not want back; some things you may realise you missed.

A specific note. If you started your antidepressant during a period of grief that was never fully processed, coming off may bring some of that grief forward in a form that feels overdue. This is not a complication. It is, arguably, part of what tapering can allow. If it feels overwhelming, a good therapist is a valuable ally. If it feels manageable, letting it move through you at its own pace is often what it needs.

> **Important Point:** *The taper is not just a chemical event. It is a re-encounter with the emotional range your drug was smoothing. Some of that range will be welcome. Some will need working through. Both are normal.*

The pull toward self-management strategies that make things worse

During the difficult weeks, the pull toward strategies that produce short-term relief but long-term worsening can be strong. Alcohol is the most common. A glass of wine in the evening may feel like the only thing softening the edges. Two glasses may feel like more relief. Over a few weeks, alcohol interferes with sleep architecture, worsens mood, and produces its own withdrawal effects the following day.

Similar patterns can develop with cannabis (which has its own withdrawal profile), with over-the-counter sleep aids used more frequently than intended, with caffeine used to compensate for poor sleep, and with prescribed benzodiazepines used more often than prescribed. None of these substances is inherently bad. All of them, used as a coping strategy during a taper, tend to compound problems rather than solve them.

If you notice a pattern developing, name it to your prescriber or to a trusted person. There is no shame in noticing it. The shame is in letting it grow while pretending it is not happening.

The pull toward other things that help

The strategies that tend to help during a taper are the ones that most patients already know about and often struggle to actually do. Movement, in whatever form is possible, most days. Time outside, ideally in daylight, most days. Contact with other humans, in whatever form your energy allows. Adequate protein and a reasonable range of nutrients. Water. Music that supports rather than agitates you. Whatever creative activity you have that quiets the front of your mind.

None of these is a cure for withdrawal. All of them are supportive practices that give your nervous system what it needs to do its adjustment work. On the good days, they compound. On the bad days, they are the difference between a hard day and a much worse one.

The trap is treating them as another performance requirement, another way to fail. They are not that. They are what you can do, at whatever scale you can do them, on the day you have. Ten minutes of walking on a bad day is better than an hour on a day that never comes.

Setbacks that are not the taper's fault

At some point during the taper, something will go wrong in your life that is not caused by the taper. Someone will get ill. A job will end. A relationship will strain. A family situation will erupt. This is what happens when a taper takes twelve or eighteen months: life keeps happening around it.

The instinct, when something goes wrong, may be to blame the taper or to abandon it. That instinct is usually not the right one. Coming off the drug did not cause the layoff or the illness or the argument. What may have happened is that the taper reduced your ordinary reserves, and the crisis has landed on a smaller buffer than usual. That is a reason to be gentler with yourself, to slow the taper or hold if you need to, and to protect the plan through the crisis. It is not usually a reason to abandon the taper entirely.

The exception is a crisis so large that you genuinely cannot maintain any focus on the taper for a while. In that case, hold at your current dose, focus on the crisis, and pick up the taper again when there is room. You have not failed. You have paused.

Ephemera worth naming

Two small things that come up often enough to mention.

Vaccinations, dental work, and minor surgeries during a taper are generally safe and do not require any change to the taper plan. If you are having a procedure that requires anaesthesia, mention the antidepressant to the anaesthetist as you would if you were on a full dose. If you have a period of acute illness (a flu, a bad cold), consider holding the taper at your current dose until you have recovered. There is no reason to add nervous system stress on top of an active infection.

Menstrual cycles, in patients who have them, may become more noticeable during the taper. Some patients find that premenstrual mood changes are more pronounced without the drug. This tends to stabilise over time. If you have specific patterns you want to track, note them in your log alongside the taper data.

The Named Principle of this chapter: a taper is a process running alongside your life, not a project done outside of it. The strategies that protect your life during the taper are the same strategies that protect your life at any difficult time. Do them at whatever scale you can, on the day you have.

In the next chapter, we look at what tends to happen after the last dose, and how to think about the first year of being off.

Chapter 16: After Zero

The last dose is a smaller moment than most people expect. There is no ceremony. The syringe goes back in the drawer, or the last half-tablet is taken, and the next morning you wake up as a person who is, for the first time in whatever number of years, no longer taking the drug.

For some readers, the days that follow will be quiet. The taper was managed carefully, the last cuts were small enough to be gentle, and the nervous system finishes its adjustment with a whisper rather than a shout. For other readers, the weeks after the last dose will bring their own patterns. Late-emerging withdrawal is real, though it is usually milder than mid-taper withdrawal. Emotional adjustment is real. Sleep may continue to shift for a while. What was in the drug's cushioning role in your life may now need to be met in other ways.

This chapter is about the first year off. It is about what to expect, what to watch for, when to reach out, and how to think about whether the outcome you have is the outcome you wanted.

The first two weeks

The first two weeks after the last dose are usually the most watched. This is when acute withdrawal, if it is going to appear, most often does. For patients who have tapered slowly and used small final cuts, this period is often quiet: the last reduction was so small that its absorption is barely noticeable.

For patients whose last cuts were slightly too large (a common finding in retrospect), some late acute withdrawal may show up here: mild brain zaps, some dizziness, sleep disturbance, occasional emotional flatness or volatility. This typically settles within one to three weeks.

If, in these first two weeks, symptoms are more than mild and are not clearly settling, contact your prescriber. A small reinstatement to your last stable dose is often the appropriate response, and it can spare you a longer, more difficult stretch. Reinstatement in the first two weeks after the last dose is generally reliable; delayed reinstatement is less predictable, as noted in Chapter 12.

Weeks three to eight

The next stretch is often quieter. Most patients settle into a new pattern of functioning without the drug, and the acute withdrawal features (if there were any) fade. Sleep may still be a bit variable. Emotional range may still be adjusting. Physical symptoms are usually gone.

This is also a stretch in which the question of relapse can appear. If you started your antidepressant for a specific condition, and if that condition is going to reappear, this is a common window for it. Chapter 11 provides the framework for distinguishing withdrawal from relapse. During weeks three to eight, that framework is worth keeping close to hand.

The general pattern to hold in mind is that acute withdrawal fades over this stretch while relapse, if it occurs, is more likely to be gradual and to look like the original condition. Late-emerging withdrawal that appears in this stretch tends to include some of the distinctive physical or sensory features rather than being purely mood-based.

For most patients, this is a period of increasing stability. If it is not, use the framework in Chapters 11 and 12 to decide what to do next.

Months two to six

The middle of the first year off is, for most patients, the settling period. Sleep normalises. Emotional range fills back in. Any lingering physical symptoms usually resolve. What tends to remain is the work of relearning how to live without the drug.

Some patients discover, in this period, that the drug had been carrying more of their life than they realised. Something that felt manageable while medicated may feel harder now, not because the drug was doing something magic, but because it was smoothing an edge they now have to face directly. This is not a failure of the taper. It is the return of an emotional signal.

The right response is not usually to go back on the drug. The right response is often to work with the signal. This may mean therapy, if you are not already in it. It may mean lifestyle adjustments. It may mean addressing a situation you had been carrying medicated. It may mean giving yourself more time.

Some patients find that they want to keep taking care of their nervous system in ways they had let slide during their years on the drug. Regular sleep. Regular movement. Regular connection. Some patients find that certain foods, certain patterns of alcohol use, or certain kinds of stress hit them harder off the drug than on. Learning what your nervous system needs, in this new configuration, is part of the first year's work.

Months six to twelve

By the second half of the first year, most patients have a clear sense of how being off the drug is working for them. Some are unequivocally glad they came off. Some have a mixed picture. A small minority have decided that the drug was serving a purpose they now miss, and are considering whether to go back on it, either at a lower dose than before or at the original dose.

Any of these outcomes is legitimate.

If you are unequivocally glad you came off, protect what you have. Keep the sleep patterns, the movement, the connection. Notice what has come back that you missed. Notice what has come back that you had not expected.

If your picture is mixed, take stock. What is working better? What is working worse? Are the harder things something you can work with (through therapy, through practice, through time), or are they signalling something that the drug was actually helping with?

If you are considering going back on the drug, this is a decision to make with your prescriber and, if possible, with a therapist who knows you well. It is not a failure of the taper. Sometimes coming off is the right thing to do; sometimes going back on is also the right thing to do. Both can be right for the same person at different times. What matters is that the decision is made deliberately, with clear eyes, on the basis of the picture in front of you now.

When to be alert for late-emerging problems

For a small proportion of patients, late-emerging withdrawal appears not in the first weeks or months but later, sometimes at three months, sometimes at six, sometimes further out. This pattern is less common than early-emerging withdrawal but is documented.

Signs to watch for include: physical or sensory symptoms that are new and distinctive (persistent tinnitus, visual disturbances, sexual dysfunction); persistent sleep disruption that does not respond to sleep supports; emotional flattening or blunting that persists beyond the first few months and does not resolve; cognitive changes that persist.

If these appear, they warrant a conversation with your prescriber. Chapter 13 covers the current understanding of protracted withdrawal, which is where such symptoms may fit.

The clinical response depends on the pattern and on how long since the last dose.

The specific question of sexual function

Sexual side effects are among the most commonly reported effects of long-term antidepressant use, and they can persist for some patients after the drug is stopped. Post-SSRI sexual dysfunction, as a specific syndrome, has been recognised in the clinical literature and is now a subject of active research. It is not universal, and it is not the outcome most patients experience, but it is real for those who develop it.

If you find, after stopping, that sexual function has not returned in the way you expected, this is worth raising with your prescriber. Some clinicians are more familiar with this than others, and referral to a specialist may be useful. Peer communities specifically for post-SSRI sexual dysfunction exist and are one route to information and support.

This book is not the definitive resource for post-SSRI sexual dysfunction. Other resources exist, including a specialist volume in the consumer clinical guide series that this book is part of, focused specifically on this syndrome. If this is your situation, seek out those resources.

The question of whether to have a plan for the future

Some patients, having successfully come off, want a plan for what to do if the original condition returns. Others prefer to cross that bridge if and when it comes.

If you want a plan, one reasonable version is this. If, at any point in the future, you find yourself experiencing symptoms that resemble the condition for which you originally took the drug, and if those symptoms are affecting your functioning, you will contact your prescriber for a conversation. That conversation may result in a period of watchful waiting, in a course of therapy, in resuming the drug at a lower dose than before, or in trying a different treatment. You do not have to know now what you would do. You need to know that you would seek advice.

Some patients find it useful to write down, briefly, what warning signs to watch for and who they would contact. This is not a plan for failure. It is a plan that means that if the situation ever arises, you are not making decisions from a compromised state without preparation.

What you have learned

By the end of the first year off, most patients have learned things they did not know when they started, and some of those things are worth naming.

You have learned what your unmedicated emotional range feels like, or you have relearned what you had partially forgotten. Some of that range is what you were hoping for. Some may have been unexpected.

You have learned what your nervous system needs to stay regulated without the drug. Sleep, movement, connection, food, light. You have learned which of these you had let slide during your medicated years, and which of these you are willing to keep prioritising now.

You have learned what your prescriber-patient partnership looks like when it works, and possibly what it looks like when it does not. You have learned to advocate for yourself in a clinical setting, using specific language and specific evidence, rather than hoping the clinician will guess what you need.

You have learned that difficult stretches pass, that patterns can be read, and that a log is worth keeping. You have learned that most bad days are not verdicts.

You have learned that coming off a long-term antidepressant is possible, at a pace your nervous system can follow, if you plan it carefully, choose your partners well, and give it the time it needs.

A note if this chapter has arrived at a hard moment

Some readers will have reached this chapter still in the middle of a difficult taper, or in a protracted state, or having reinstated after an attempt that did not go as planned. If that is you, and if reading a chapter about a settled first year off is difficult, I understand.

You have not failed. What you have is a hard piece of a longer story. Most people who taper an antidepressant reach some version of what this chapter describes, though the timeframe is not always what they hoped. Some reach a settled first year off after two or three attempts. Some reach it after a difficult first year that got easier over time. Some find that the right outcome for them is a lower dose than they were on, held stably, rather than zero.

Where you are now is not necessarily where you will be. The information in this book is for the whole trajectory, not just for the easy parts. If you need to reread Chapter 12 on holds and reinstatement, or Chapter 13 on protracted withdrawal, or Chapter 14 on the conversation with your prescriber, do that. If you need to talk to someone, please reach out.

The Named Principle of this chapter: the first year off is a settling year, not a testing year. What you learned during the taper about your nervous system, your prescriber, and yourself is now the material you carry forward, and it belongs to you regardless of what shape the year ahead takes.

The last chapter is a short conclusion, which brings the strands together.

Conclusion: What You Have Now That You Did Not Have Before

The book is nearly over. Before you close it, I want to name what you have, so that when you put it down and go on with your life, you go on with the strands gathered.

You have a mental model of what your drug is doing in your body, and why coming off it is not the same as never having started. You know which drug family yours belongs to. You know its half-life. You know why that half-life matters. You know that the drug's therapeutic action and its withdrawal profile are two different things, even though they are hosted by the same molecule.

You have precise language for the four states that are usually shuffled together. Physical dependence. Addiction. Withdrawal. Relapse. You know that these words describe different phenomena, that they are not interchangeable, and that using the right word can change the direction of the plan.

You have a pharmacological picture of why the standard advice fails so often, and why a hyperbolic taper works better. You know that receptor occupancy does not scale linearly with dose, that equal cuts in milligrams do not produce equal cuts in effect, and that reductions must get smaller as the dose gets smaller if the taper is to be evenly paced at the receptor. You know that this is not a controversial claim; it is the current mainstream view in the deprescribing literature.

You have a way to check whether now is the right time for you to start. You have questions to ask about your housing, your relationships, your work, the support around you, and your reasons for wanting to come off. You know that postponing when the conditions are wrong is not weakness. You know that starting when the conditions are right is what makes a difference.

You have a plan. Five decisions: initial reduction size, interval, pattern, goal, review points. You have a template to draft it. You know what to bring to your prescriber.

You have a formulation strategy. Licensed liquids, compounded liquids, bead counting, tapering strips, splitting, water titration, cross-tapering. You know which of these fits your specific drug, and you know that solving the formulation question is what makes the plan implementable.

You have a specific schedule for your specific drug, from Chapter 7, 8, or 9. You know it is a starting point, not a prescription, and that it will need to be adjusted in conversation with your prescriber.

You have a symptom map. You know what to expect. You know what warrants urgent attention. You know that most withdrawal symptoms are unpleasant but not dangerous, and that the ones that are dangerous have specific patterns you can recognise.

You have a framework for the most consequential judgement of any taper: is this withdrawal, or is it relapse? Four dimensions. Timing, symptom pattern, response to reinstatement, comparison with baseline. You know how to work through them and when a reinstatement trial is the right next step.

You have decision rules for the moments that will come up. Hold. Slow. Reinstate. You know when each is appropriate, how to do each in practice, and why none of them is a failure.

You have an honest picture of protracted withdrawal. You know it is real and uncommon. You know what it can look like, who is at higher risk, what tends to help and what does not, and when to seek specialist support. If you turn out to be in that territory, you know you are not alone and you are not permanently broken.

You have scripts for the conversation with your prescriber. Five of them, for the specific situations that come up most often. You know how to describe symptoms in clinical language. You know how to name your interpretation. You know how to invite their view. You know that this is a negotiation between partners, and you know what to do if the partnership is not working.

You have a plan for the rest of your life while the taper is happening. Sleep. Work. Family. Emotional reappearance. The pull toward things that make it harder and the pull toward things that make it easier. You know that the strategies that protect life during a taper are the same strategies that protect life at any difficult time, and you know that you can do them at whatever scale you can do them on the day you have.

You have a picture of the first year after zero. The two weeks. The next six weeks. The middle months. The end of the year. You know when to be alert for late-emerging problems. You know that the first year is a settling year, and that what you learned during the taper is now the material you carry forward.

That is what you have.

You did not have most of it a few hundred pages ago. You have it now. It is not nothing. It is enough, in my experience, to give a well-planned taper a very good chance of success. It is enough, if things go differently, to give you a framework for figuring out what to do next.

The last thing I want to say is this. Coming off an antidepressant, in the year I am writing this book, is a different undertaking from what it was ten or twenty years ago. What you are attempting is now supported by a body of clinical knowledge and by a small but growing community of clinicians and researchers who understand what tapering actually requires. You are not the first to attempt it, and you will not be the last. What you are doing is being done by many people, at their own pace, in their own way, all over the world, right now.

If it takes longer than you hoped, that is fine. If it needs to be adjusted, that is fine. If you decide, at some point, that a lower stable dose is your right outcome rather than zero, that is fine. If, months from now, you find yourself thinking of the drug not as an enemy or a friend but as a tool that once had a use, that is a good place to arrive at.

Whatever the shape of your particular taper, I wish you a settled nervous system, a supportive prescriber, and the sleep you need.

Stella Marion Kaufman

Appendix A: The Taper Plan Worksheet

This worksheet gives you a template for drafting the plan you will bring to your prescriber. Copy it into a notebook or a document, fill in your specifics, and use it as a starting point for the conversation.

Section one: your drug profile.

Drug name (generic): _______

Drug name (brand): _______

Current dose: _______ mg

Formulation: tablet / capsule / liquid / other _______

Standard release or extended release: _______

Length of time on this drug: _______ years / months

Any past attempts to come off, and what happened: _______

Reason for wanting to come off now: _______

Section two: your five decisions.

Decision one, initial reduction size: 25% / 10% / 5% (circle one, based on Chapter 5 guidance).

Decision two, reduction interval: minimum _______ weeks between reductions.

Decision three, pattern: fixed-percentage cuts / example schedule from Chapter 7, 8, or 9 / hybrid.

Decision four, goal: zero / a specific lower dose of _______ mg.

Decision five, review points: at _______ months, at _______ months, at _______ months, and after any hold longer than _______ weeks.

Section three: your formulation strategy.

How will you achieve the smaller doses when they come? Circle all that apply.

Standard tablets from pharmacy.

Split tablets using a pill cutter.

Licensed liquid from pharmacy.

Compounded liquid from compounding pharmacy.

Bead counting from extended-release capsules.

Tapering strips.

Other: _______

Compounding pharmacy contact if using: _______

Section four: your support.

Prescriber name and contact: _______

Anyone at home who knows you are doing this: _______

Anyone outside home who knows: _______

Emergency plan if things get worse: _______

Section five: your first three months, sketched.

Month one, starting dose: _______ mg. First planned reduction to: _______ mg on approximately _______ (date).

Month two, planned reduction to: _______ mg on approximately _______ (date), or hold if not yet stable.

Month three, planned reduction to: _______ mg on approximately _______ (date), or hold if not yet stable.

First review point: _______ (date).

Draft this worksheet before your first appointment. Bring it with you. Expect it to be adjusted in conversation. The version you leave the appointment with is the version to start.

Appendix B: The Symptom-Tracking Log

This log gives you a template for tracking your symptoms across the taper. Keep it daily. It is the single most useful data you will bring to any appointment.

You can keep it in a paper diary, in a spreadsheet, or in a notes app. What matters is consistency, not format.

Daily entry template.

Date: _______

Day of taper: _______

Current dose: _______ mg

Days since last reduction: _______

Sleep quality, 1 (very poor) to 5 (excellent): _______

Sleep duration, hours: _______

Mood, 1 (very low) to 5 (very good): _______

Anxiety, 1 (none) to 5 (severe): _______

Physical symptoms today, mark any that apply.

Dizziness: yes / no

Brain zaps: yes / no

Headache: yes / no

Nausea or gastrointestinal upset: yes / no

Fatigue: yes / no

Muscle aches: yes / no

Sensory changes (light or sound sensitivity, other): yes / no

Sensory persistence pattern noticed: yes / no

Gait instability: yes / no

Sleep symptoms today, mark any that apply.

Difficulty falling asleep: yes / no

Night wakings: yes / no

Vivid dreams: yes / no

Early morning waking: yes / no

Emotional symptoms today, mark any that apply.

Heightened anxiety: yes / no

Tearfulness: yes / no

Irritability: yes / no

Emotional volatility: yes / no

Rage or intense anger: yes / no

Low mood: yes / no

Cognitive symptoms today, mark any that apply.

Brain fog: yes / no

Concentration difficulties: yes / no

Depersonalisation or derealisation: yes / no

Memory blips: yes / no

Notes on the day, one line: _______

Weekly review, once a week: what pattern have I noticed this week compared with last week? _______

Monthly review, once a month: is my overall trajectory improving, stable, or worsening? _______

Bring this log to every appointment. Even the sections your prescriber does not directly discuss are useful for your own tracking. A pattern that is invisible day by day often becomes clear across weeks.

Appendix C: Withdrawal or Relapse, The Decision Aid

Use this aid when you are trying to work out whether current symptoms are withdrawal, relapse, or a mixed picture.

Question one, timing. When did the current symptoms start?

Within days to two weeks of a dose reduction or the final dose: points to withdrawal.

Two to six weeks after a stable state was reached: could be either; consider other dimensions.

Six weeks or more after a stable state was reached, with gradual emergence: points to relapse.

Question two, symptom pattern. What symptoms are present?

Physical or sensory symptoms that were not part of the original condition (brain zaps, dizziness, sensory changes, gait instability): points to withdrawal.

A mix of physical and mood symptoms: could be either.

Symptoms that closely resemble the original condition (depression pattern, panic pattern, anxiety pattern) without new physical features: points to relapse.

Question three, response to reinstatement. If a small reinstatement has been tried, what happened?

Substantial improvement within a few days to a week: strongly points to withdrawal.

No improvement, or improvement only over weeks with dose adjustment: points to relapse.

Reinstatement not yet tried: this dimension is unanswered.

Question four, comparison with baseline. Does what you are feeling now resemble what you were feeling before you started the drug?

No, this feels different: points to withdrawal.

Some yes, some no: mixed picture.

Yes, this feels very like the state I was in before I started: points to relapse.

Scoring, informally.

If three or more dimensions point to withdrawal: proceed on that basis. Discuss with your prescriber. Options are hold, slow, or reinstate as per Chapter 12.

If three or more dimensions point to relapse: proceed on that basis. Discuss with your prescriber. Options include reinstating the drug, trying a different medication, adding therapy, or adding non-drug supports.

If the picture is mixed: a reinstatement trial is often the most useful next step. Discuss with your prescriber. Reinstate to your last stable dose, hold for two to three weeks, and observe. Rapid improvement supports withdrawal; slow or partial improvement supports relapse; no change supports something else that will need further assessment.

If the picture includes thoughts of self-harm or suicide, whichever it turns out to be, treat it as urgent. Reinstate to a stable dose without waiting. Contact your prescriber. Reach for crisis support if needed (988 in the US, Samaritans 116 123 or NHS 111 in the UK, local equivalents elsewhere). You do not have to figure out the diagnosis before you get help.

Appendix D: Bead-Counting Worksheet, With A Venlafaxine Worked Example

This appendix is for readers using bead counting from extended-release capsules (venlafaxine or duloxetine) to achieve small dose reductions. Do not use this method without your prescriber's knowledge.

Step one. Determine the number of beads in one capsule. This varies slightly by manufacturer, so do it once for the capsule you are actually using. Open one capsule carefully over a clean surface. Count all the beads. Alternatively, if you have access to a fine kitchen scale (precision to 0.001 g is ideal), weigh the beads and divide by the milligram strength to get an approximate per-bead weight.

Example: a 75 mg venlafaxine XR capsule is opened. Approximately 300 beads are counted. Each bead is approximately 0.25 mg.

Step two. Determine your current daily dose in beads. If you are currently taking 75 mg, that is 300 beads. If you are currently taking 37.5 mg, that is 150 beads.

Step three. Determine the number of beads to remove for the next reduction.

For a 10% reduction, remove 10% of the beads.

From 300 beads (75 mg): remove 30 beads. Take 270 beads (approximately 67.5 mg).

From 270 beads (67.5 mg): remove 27 beads. Take 243 beads (approximately 60.75 mg).

For a 5% reduction, remove 5% of the beads.

From 150 beads (37.5 mg): remove approximately 7 or 8 beads. Take approximately 142 to 143 beads (approximately 35.5 mg).

Step four. Deliver the dose. The beads are designed to be swallowed whole. Do not crush or chew them. Some patients place the counted beads into an empty gelatin capsule (available inexpensively from most compounding pharmacies) so that they can be swallowed as a single capsule. Others sprinkle them onto a spoonful of soft food that is swallowed immediately.

Step five. Store consistently. If you are counting beads for multiple days, ideally count each day's dose freshly rather than storing beads outside the capsule, since the coating on some beads may be affected by air exposure. Alternatively, count all your beads once, place each daily dose into a separate empty capsule, and store the prepared capsules in a dry container away from heat and light.

Notes on precision. Bead-based dosing is not as precise as a compounded liquid. Manufacturer beads vary slightly in weight, and counting introduces small errors. For most patients, this level of precision is adequate. If you are highly sensitive and small variations produce noticeable symptoms, consider switching to a compounded liquid at the mid or lower part of the taper.

Notes on safety. Not all capsules are designed to be opened. Do not open enteric-coated capsules or capsules that specifically state they should not be split or opened. If in doubt, ask your pharmacist about the specific product you have. Duloxetine capsules contain enteric-coated pellets that must be swallowed intact; do not chew them.

Appendix E: For Your Prescriber, One Page

This appendix is designed to be photocopied or printed as a single page and handed to your prescriber. It summarises the evidence base for the tapering approach in this book. It is deliberately compact.

To the prescriber.

Your patient is planning a taper of an SSRI, SNRI, mirtazapine, or trazodone using a hyperbolic reduction pattern. This page summarises the evidence supporting this approach.

The pharmacological rationale. Serotonin transporter occupancy has been shown, in positron emission tomography studies, to follow a hyperbolic dose-occupancy relationship for SSRIs. Equal reductions in milligrams do not produce equal reductions in receptor occupancy: low-dose reductions produce disproportionately large changes in effect at the receptor. The clinical implication is that reductions in milligrams should get smaller as the dose gets smaller, in order to produce even reductions in effect at the receptor across the taper. This is now the mainstream view in the deprescribing literature.

The clinical rationale for a slow taper. Withdrawal syndromes from SSRIs, SNRIs, mirtazapine, and trazodone are now well-documented and can be severe and prolonged in a subset of patients, particularly those with long-term exposure. Rapid tapers (weeks) are associated with higher rates of withdrawal-related distress and higher rates of failed discontinuation than slow tapers (months to a year or more). A slow taper does not guarantee absence of withdrawal, but it substantially reduces both the severity and the persistence.

Key references. Horowitz M A, Taylor D M (2019), "Tapering of SSRI treatment to mitigate withdrawal symptoms," The Lancet Psychiatry 6(6), 538 to 546. Horowitz M A, Taylor D M (2024), Deprescribing guidelines for psychiatric medications, second edition (specific title varies by publication; the general clinical framework is well-established in the current literature). Fava G A, Belaise C (2018) and related work on antidepressant discontinuation syndrome. Hengartner M P et al (2020), on protracted withdrawal presentation and duration. Recent systematic reviews on post-acute withdrawal syndromes (2025 update).

The role of the prescriber. Successful tapers depend critically on the prescriber's willingness to support hyperbolic schedules, to prescribe liquid formulations or compounded formulations where standard tablets do not deliver the required dose, and to distinguish withdrawal from relapse when new symptoms emerge. Standard 25% reductions over four weeks are inconsistent with the current evidence base for most long-term users of most drugs in this book.

If your patient is presenting new symptoms after a dose reduction, please consider withdrawal as a differential diagnosis alongside relapse. Timing (rapid onset after reduction), symptom pattern (physical and sensory symptoms not part of the original condition), and response to reinstatement (rapid improvement on returning to a previous stable dose) are the standard diagnostic features. Where the picture is ambiguous, a small reinstatement trial provides both symptomatic relief and diagnostic information.

Thank you for supporting your patient through this process.

Appendix F: Support Resources By Country

The resources listed here are current at the time of writing. Availability and contact details may change; please verify before use.

Urgent mental health support

United States. National Suicide and Crisis Lifeline: call or text 988. This service is available 24 hours a day, seven days a week.

United Kingdom and Republic of Ireland. Samaritans: call 116 123. This service is available 24 hours a day. NHS 111 is also available for urgent mental health advice, and NHS 111 Option 2 in some areas is a dedicated mental health line.

Canada. Call or text 988 for the Suicide Crisis Helpline.

Australia. Lifeline: 13 11 14. Available 24 hours a day.

New Zealand. Need to Talk: call or text 1737. Lifeline Aotearoa: 0800 543 354.

Other countries. The International Association for Suicide Prevention maintains a directory of crisis lines by country, searchable online. If you are in a country not listed here, look for your national equivalent.

If you or someone with you is in immediate physical danger, contact your local emergency service (911 in the US and Canada, 999 in the UK and Ireland, 000 in Australia, 111 in New Zealand, 112 in most of Europe).

Antidepressant deprescribing information and peer support

Surviving Antidepressants. A peer-led online forum with a large archive of tapering experiences, symptom descriptions, and general information. Not a substitute for medical care, but a widely used community resource.

Inner Compass Initiative. A US-based organisation providing information and community support around psychiatric drug withdrawal.

Council for Evidence-based Psychiatry. A UK-based organisation focused on prescribing and deprescribing information.

Outro Health. A US-based clinical service offering guided taper support with prescribing clinicians familiar with hyperbolic tapering.

Post-SSRI sexual dysfunction

The PSSD Network. A patient-led organisation for those experiencing persistent sexual dysfunction after stopping antidepressants. Provides information and community support.

Rxisk.org. A patient-facing site with information about post-SSRI sexual dysfunction and other persistent effects of psychiatric medications.

For clinicians

The current international clinical literature on deprescribing includes ongoing publications from academic researchers and clinical services. Prescribers seeking to develop deprescribing competence may consider training with organisations such as the International Institute for Psychiatric Drug Withdrawal, or specialist units at teaching hospitals with an interest in deprescribing.

For families and partners

Family and partner support during a taper is often less discussed than patient support. If you are a family member or partner, the resources listed above are also useful for you, particularly the peer communities where partners and family members share their experiences.

The books "Coming Off Antidepressants" and other consumer clinical guides in the series that includes this book contain further reading for families and partners specifically.

Appendix G: Glossary

Anticholinergic. Refers to substances or effects that block the action of the neurotransmitter acetylcholine. Some antidepressants, particularly paroxetine, have anticholinergic effects that can produce symptoms such as dry mouth, blurred vision, constipation, and urinary retention. Anticholinergic rebound during withdrawal produces the opposite pattern.

Brain zap. A brief, shock-like sensation in the head, often described as a jolt of electricity, sometimes accompanied by a buzzing sound. Common in withdrawal from SSRIs and SNRIs, particularly paroxetine and venlafaxine. Not dangerous; not a seizure. Typically triggered by eye movement, head turning, or fatigue.

Compounding pharmacy. A pharmacy that prepares medications individually to specific formulations, rather than dispensing pre-manufactured tablets. Can produce custom-concentration liquids and non-standard tablet doses. Availability and regulation vary by country.

Depersonalisation. The subjective experience of feeling detached from one's own body or self, as if watching oneself from outside. Can occur during withdrawal from SSRIs and SNRIs. Usually time-limited.

Derealisation. The subjective experience of the external world feeling unreal, dreamlike, or distant. Related to depersonalisation and often accompanies it during withdrawal.

Discontinuation syndrome. A term used in older clinical literature to describe symptoms occurring when antidepressants are stopped. Current literature generally uses "withdrawal" instead, since the phenomenon is a withdrawal syndrome in the physiological sense.

Extended release. A pharmaceutical formulation designed to release its active ingredient slowly over an extended period, typically twelve to twenty-four hours. Often abbreviated XR, ER, or SR (slow release). Some extended-release formulations cannot be split or crushed.

Fluoxetine bridge. A tapering technique in which a patient is switched from a short-half-life antidepressant (typically paroxetine or venlafaxine) to fluoxetine, and then the fluoxetine is tapered. Uses fluoxetine's very long half-life to cushion the withdrawal process.

Half-life. The time it takes for the concentration of a drug in the body to decrease by half after intake ends. Determines how quickly a drug leaves the system after a dose is missed or reduced. Short half-lives are associated with more difficult tapers.

Hyperbolic tapering. A tapering approach in which the size of dose reductions decreases as the dose decreases, producing approximately equal reductions in receptor occupancy at each step rather than equal reductions in milligrams. The current standard approach for most antidepressant tapers.

Muscarinic receptor. A receptor for the neurotransmitter acetylcholine. Paroxetine, among a few antidepressants in this book, has activity at muscarinic receptors, which contributes to its anticholinergic side effect profile and to specific withdrawal features.

Norfluoxetine. The active metabolite of fluoxetine. Has a very long half-life (one to two weeks), which contributes to fluoxetine's unique tapering profile.

Norepinephrine. A neurotransmitter involved in alertness, arousal, and the stress response. Also known as noradrenaline in some countries. Targeted by SNRIs and by mirtazapine's indirect mechanism.

Physical dependence. A physiological state in which the body has adapted to the ongoing presence of a substance and would react in some way if the substance were suddenly removed. Distinct from addiction.

Post-acute withdrawal syndrome (PAWS). A term borrowed from the substance-use literature and used by some authors to describe protracted antidepressant withdrawal. Not universally adopted for antidepressants.

Post-SSRI sexual dysfunction (PSSD). A syndrome of persistent sexual dysfunction following the use of SSRIs, which can continue after the drug is stopped. Recognised in the clinical literature and the subject of ongoing research.

Protracted withdrawal. A withdrawal syndrome that persists for months to years after the drug has been stopped. Uncommon but documented. Discussed in Chapter 13.

Receptor occupancy. The proportion of a receptor population that is bound by a drug at a given moment. For SSRIs, receptor occupancy at the serotonin transporter follows a hyperbolic relationship with dose.

Reinstatement. The practice of returning to a previous dose after a reduction has produced difficult symptoms. Discussed in Chapter 12.

Selective serotonin reuptake inhibitor (SSRI). A class of antidepressant that primarily blocks the reuptake of serotonin at the synapse. Includes sertraline, escitalopram, citalopram, fluoxetine, and paroxetine.

Serotonin and norepinephrine reuptake inhibitor (SNRI). A class of antidepressant that blocks the reuptake of both serotonin and norepinephrine. Includes venlafaxine, duloxetine, and desvenlafaxine.

Tapering strip. A manufactured product in which each day's dose is slightly smaller than the previous day's, packaged in a sequential strip. Available in some countries but not all.

Water titration. The practice of dissolving a tablet in a known volume of water to achieve small custom doses. Precision varies by drug; not universally recommended.

Withdrawal. The set of symptoms that emerges when a substance to which the body has become physically dependent is reduced or removed. Distinct from addiction and from relapse.

Appendix H: Further Reading and Sources

The list below is a curated set of sources that supported the writing of this book. The full list of citations is in the References section that follows. This appendix is a shorter list intended for readers who want to read further.

For an accessible, patient-facing introduction to the case for hyperbolic tapering, Horowitz and Taylor's 2019 paper in The Lancet Psychiatry ("Tapering of SSRI treatment to mitigate withdrawal symptoms") is the foundational article. It is written for clinicians but is readable by non-specialists.

For a general clinical framework, the current deprescribing literature from Horowitz, Taylor, and their collaborators is the most widely cited body of work in the field. The 2024 clinical guidance published in this area draws together the receptor-occupancy science, the withdrawal literature, and the practical taper schedules for the drugs covered in this book. Interested readers can find the current versions through medical libraries and, for some material, through the academic literature.

For the recognition of protracted withdrawal, Hengartner and colleagues' 2020 paper on the presentation and duration of protracted antidepressant withdrawal is the most systematic published survey data to date. The 2025 systematic review on post-acute withdrawal provides an updated synthesis.

For patient-reported perspectives that have shaped the field, the archive at the Surviving Antidepressants forum is unmatched as a resource of case histories. It should not be read as a substitute for medical care, but it is invaluable for understanding what tapering actually looks like from the inside for large numbers of people.

For post-SSRI sexual dysfunction specifically, the PSSD Network and Rxisk.org are the most active patient-facing resources, and the academic literature on the syndrome has grown substantially since 2018.

For the wider context of overprescribing and deprescribing of psychiatric medications, Anders Sørensen's 2024 book on withdrawing from psychiatric drugs is a broad-ranging lay-oriented resource. Joanna Moncrieff's writing on the wider case for critical psychiatry provides intellectual context, though its arguments range beyond the specific tapering focus of this book.

For readers looking for further clinical support beyond what a general prescriber can offer, specialist deprescribing clinics have begun to appear in some countries. Access varies; a psychiatric referral is often the most reliable route.

The consumer clinical guide series to which this book belongs includes other titles on adjacent topics, including sexual dysfunction after antidepressant use, coming off other psychiatric medications, and specific mental health conditions for which antidepressants are often prescribed. Readers who find this book useful may find the other titles useful as well.

Appendix I: Common Questions

These are the questions that come up most often, in clinics and in peer communities, at the various stages of a taper. They are not meant to substitute for the fuller treatment in the main chapters; they are meant to give you quick, direct answers to the questions readers ask most.

Before starting

Is it too late to come off, if I have been on the drug for many years?

No. Long-term use makes a slower taper more important, but it does not make coming off impossible. Many patients successfully come off after ten, fifteen, or twenty years on their antidepressant. The plan needs to be gentler and longer, and the formulation strategy needs to be robust, but the underlying possibility is unchanged.

Should I taper if my life is generally good and the drug seems to be helping?

That depends on why you want to come off. If you are content with your current state and the drug is producing no side effects that trouble you, staying on is a legitimate choice. If you want to see what your unmedicated baseline is like, or if a side effect is bothering you, tapering is legitimate too. There is no obligation either way. What matters is that the decision is yours and that it is made deliberately.

Can I taper without my prescriber knowing?

Please do not. Every method described in this book that reaches the small doses needed for a proper hyperbolic taper requires prescriber cooperation, either for the liquid formulation, for the compounded formulation, or for the reinstatement option if things go wrong. If your current prescriber will not support a taper, use the scripts in Chapter 14 to try to bring them along, or change prescribers. What you should not do is proceed alone.

Should I taper if I am pregnant, or planning to conceive?

This is a specific conversation to have with your obstetrician and your prescriber together. Some patients successfully taper before conception. Some remain on their antidepressant through pregnancy, because the risk of untreated illness during pregnancy is significant. There is no single right answer, and the trade-offs depend on your specific history, your specific drug, and your specific plans. What you should not do is stop the drug abruptly on discovering you are pregnant, because acute withdrawal in early pregnancy is not desirable either.

During the taper

I have missed a dose. What should I do?

If the missed dose was for a drug with a short half-life (venlafaxine, duloxetine, paroxetine), and you notice within the same day, take it as soon as you remember. If it is already close to your next scheduled dose, do not double up; skip it and continue. Missed doses on these drugs are unpleasant but not usually dangerous. Multiple missed doses in a row will produce full withdrawal.

For drugs with long half-lives (fluoxetine, and to a lesser extent sertraline and citalopram), a single missed dose is usually inconsequential. Take the next scheduled dose as normal.

Regardless of the drug, if you find yourself repeatedly missing doses, that is worth addressing. Set an alarm. Use a pill organiser. Anchor the dose to an activity you always do (brushing your teeth, first coffee). Consistency of dosing during the taper is not optional; it is what allows you to interpret what your body is doing.

I forgot to take my liquid dose but I took my tablet. What now?

If you have been switching between formulations, mid-taper confusion is real. Write down what you took and when. Do not take an additional dose to compensate. Continue with your normal schedule from the next dose. If you are unsure whether you have double-dosed, contact your prescriber or pharmacist. The general principle is that a single mistake is not usually dangerous, but a pattern of mistakes should be corrected.

I feel fine, can I move to the next reduction faster than the plan says?

Possibly, but be careful. Some patients tolerate faster tapers well; others discover the difficulty only at the smaller doses. If you are considering accelerating, discuss it with your prescriber first. If you do accelerate, do so with a small increment, not a large one, and be prepared to slow down if symptoms appear.

I feel terrible, does that mean I have to stop the taper entirely?

Almost certainly not. Feeling terrible after a reduction typically means that the reduction was too large or too soon, and the correct response is to hold, slow, or reinstate to a previous stable dose, not to abandon the whole project. Chapter 12 walks you through this decision. Discuss with your prescriber. Give yourself permission to slow down.

Should I get my serotonin levels tested?

No. Blood serotonin levels do not meaningfully reflect brain serotonin function and are not useful for tapering decisions. Similarly, there is no reliable blood test that tells you whether your withdrawal is real or how far along you are in adjusting. The best data source for your taper is your symptom log.

About symptoms

Are brain zaps dangerous?

No. They are unpleasant, sometimes distressing, and occasionally frightening the first time they occur, but they are not dangerous. They do not indicate seizure activity or brain damage. They are a specific neurological signature of certain withdrawal states and they resolve as the withdrawal resolves.

Can withdrawal cause seizures?

For the drugs in this book, seizures caused by withdrawal are rare. They are not, in most cases, a realistic concern. This is in contrast to benzodiazepine or alcohol withdrawal, which can cause seizures and which require medical supervision for that reason.

If you have a personal history of seizures, or if you have other medical conditions that affect seizure risk, this is worth mentioning to your prescriber before starting the taper. For most patients, seizure risk is not a factor.

Is emotional flatness during the taper permanent?

Usually not. Most emotional flatness during a taper resolves as the taper proceeds and the nervous system re-adjusts. In a minority of patients, emotional blunting can persist after the drug is stopped. This is discussed in Chapter 13 and is one of the presentations of protracted withdrawal.

If your emotional flatness is persistent and is affecting your life, discuss it with your prescriber. There is currently no specific pharmacological treatment for it. Time, nervous system support, and, for some patients, therapy that works with the body as well as the mind, tend to help.

I am having weird dreams. Is that normal?

Yes. Vivid, unusual, or unsettling dreams are a very common feature of antidepressant withdrawal, particularly with mirtazapine, trazodone, and the SNRIs. They typically resolve within days to weeks per reduction. If they are severely distressing or are disturbing your sleep for extended periods, mention them to your prescriber.

About specific situations

Can I drink alcohol during a taper?

You can, in moderation, but be aware that alcohol tends to worsen sleep, mood, and cognitive symptoms during a taper. It also interacts with several of the drugs in this book in ways that can make you more affected by a given amount than usual. If you are going to drink, keep the amount modest, keep it away from bedtime, and pay attention to how you feel the next day.

If you notice that alcohol is becoming a way of managing withdrawal symptoms, please name it to yourself and to someone you trust. This pattern can develop quickly and can add a second withdrawal problem on top of the first.

Can I take other medications during a taper?

Most medications for physical health conditions can be continued as normal. Some medications, particularly certain painkillers and certain migraine treatments, can interact with SSRIs or SNRIs in specific ways. If you are prescribed a new medication during your taper, mention your antidepressant to the prescriber and ask about interactions.

Over-the-counter cold and flu medications sometimes contain ingredients that interact with antidepressants. Check with your pharmacist before taking a new one.

Can I fly during a taper?

Yes, generally. Flying does not affect the taper itself. Time zone changes may temporarily disrupt sleep and dose timing; try to take your dose at the same local time as you were taking it before the flight (or the same UTC time, whichever your prescriber recommends). Long-haul flights sometimes coincide with a bad reaction to the previous week's reduction; if you have a big trip coming, consider holding at your current dose through the trip and resuming reductions after you return.

Can I have surgery during a taper?

Usually yes. Mention your current dose and the taper plan to the anaesthetist and surgical team. Some clinicians will recommend holding at your current dose through the peri-operative period rather than making a reduction close to surgery, which is sensible.

Should I have therapy during a taper?

If you already have a therapist, keep going. If you do not, and if your budget and access allow, therapy during a taper is often useful. What tends to be most helpful is a therapist who is comfortable with the physical and emotional realities of nervous system dysregulation and who does not interpret every difficult day as a psychological problem. Body-based, trauma-informed, and pace-sensitive approaches are often mentioned by patients as helpful.

If you cannot access private therapy, low-cost options exist in many countries. Group therapy, peer support, and structured self-help materials can also provide some of the support that individual therapy offers.

After finishing

How will I know I am fully recovered?

Full recovery, for most patients, means several months of stable functioning off the drug, with no persistent physical, sensory, or cognitive symptoms and with an emotional range that feels normal to you. There is no single test or milestone. The general answer is that if you have been off the drug for six to twelve months and you feel like yourself, the taper is completed and recovery is well established.

Can I ever go back on if I need to?

Yes. If, at some future point, the condition for which you originally took the drug returns, or a different condition emerges, restarting an antidepressant is a legitimate option to discuss with your prescriber. The successful taper is not spoiled by a subsequent decision to go back on. It is a piece of information you had that year, and if the situation later changes, your options are open.

Some patients specifically ask whether they will need a slower titration up if they restart. Usually not, unless you had significant tolerance issues. Restarting is generally straightforward. Whether to restart at all is the question that matters, not whether you can.

Will my body ever be the same as before I started?

For most patients, yes, in the sense that ordinary functioning returns. Some patients notice that they are slightly more sensitive to certain things than they were before (alcohol, poor sleep, stress), and this may be a permanent feature of a nervous system that has been through both the drug and the taper. This is usually manageable and, for most people, is not a significant restriction.

A minority of patients continue to notice some persistent effects, particularly around emotional range or sexual function, and this is the terrain covered by Chapter 13 and the further reading in Appendix H.

For most patients, most of the time, life after the taper is not a diminished version of life before. It is life as it is now, with what you learned along the way.

Appendix J: Notes for Family and Partners

This appendix is for the person supporting a family member or partner through a taper. If that is you, read this before the taper starts if possible. If the taper is already underway, read it now.

What is actually happening

Your person is coming off a medication that has been part of their neurochemistry for months or years. The process is designed to be slow and controlled, and most tapers proceed without significant crisis. But even a well-planned taper can produce, at various points, days or weeks when your person's nervous system is more reactive than usual, their sleep is disturbed, their emotional range is more variable, and their capacity to absorb ordinary life stressors is temporarily reduced.

This is not a mental health crisis. It is not a return of their original condition (usually). It is a physiological adjustment to a lower level of a drug their body had adapted to.

What they need from you is not, in most cases, to fix anything. What they need is understanding, patience, and specific practical support during the harder stretches. This appendix names what that looks like.

What to expect over the course of the taper

The overall pattern of a taper is one of periods of relative stability separated by shorter periods of adjustment. In the days after each dose reduction, symptoms may emerge (physical, sensory, sleep, emotional, or cognitive). These typically peak within one to two weeks and then settle. Between reductions, your person is often close to their normal self.

Not every reduction will produce difficulty. Some pass with little disturbance. Others produce a rougher stretch. The pattern is not fully predictable, but it tends to become more manageable as both of you learn what to expect.

Your person may also, at some point during the taper, experience a return of feelings they had not had for a long time. This can be positive (tears at a piece of music, laughter that surprises them, grief they had partially forgotten). It can also be disorienting. For many patients, this emotional reappearance is one of the reasons they wanted to come off in the first place. For others, it is uncomfortable and takes some getting used to.

What tends to help

The single most useful thing you can do is to not take their variability personally. If they are short with you after a reduction, it is not because they are angry with you. If they seem distant or preoccupied, it is not because they have lost interest in you. This is your person having a rough day in the specific way that antidepressant withdrawal produces. It will pass.

The second most useful thing is to help protect the routines that stabilise their nervous system. Consistent bedtimes. Consistent mealtimes. Time outside, particularly in the morning. Moderate movement. Reduced alcohol and caffeine, at least during the harder weeks. These are not lifestyle prescriptions from you to them; they are shared conditions in the household that make everything easier.

The third useful thing is to be a partner in the practical work of the taper. This might mean going to appointments with them if that helps. It might mean helping them keep the symptom log by reminding them of things they might otherwise forget. It might mean handling more of the household load during the hardest weeks and less during the settled ones. It might mean simply being someone they can say "today is a rough day" to, without them having to explain further.

What to watch for

Most withdrawal patterns do not require you to intervene. Some do. Signs that your person may need additional support, and that you should encourage them to reach out to their prescriber or crisis line, include:

Any expression of thoughts about self-harm or ending life that is more than fleeting. If they mention this, take it seriously. Ask them to contact their prescriber. If they will not, ask whether you can help them do it. If they are in immediate distress, help them access urgent crisis support.

Severe insomnia over several nights. If they have not slept for two or three nights in a row, this is worth a call to their prescriber.

Marked functional collapse. If they cannot get out of bed, cannot eat, cannot manage basic self-care, and this is not improving day by day, they need to reach out for support.

Symptoms that seem physically unusual (chest pain, seizure-like activity, difficulty breathing) require immediate medical assessment.

The general principle is that you are not their therapist and you are not their prescriber. You do not have to diagnose what is happening. You do have to notice when things seem to be more than they can manage alone and to help them access help.

What not to do

Do not press them to speed up the taper because it is inconvenient. The taper is on the pace their nervous system can absorb. Trying to shorten it usually lengthens the whole process by producing a failed attempt and a reinstatement.

Do not press them to slow down or abandon the taper because you find their variability difficult. If you have concerns, name them, and let them decide with their prescriber what to do. Their taper is their decision.

Do not assume that a difficult day means the whole plan is failing. Look at the pattern over weeks, not days. Bad days pass. Weeks of steadily worsening symptoms are a different matter and warrant attention.

Do not compare their experience with anyone else's. Every nervous system is different. What was easy for one person may be hard for another, and the reverse.

Do not use their taper as ammunition in a disagreement. If they are irritable and short with you, that is a moment for patience, not for accusations about their behaviour. This is one of the specific ways that tapers can strain relationships, and it is worth noticing when you catch yourself heading toward it.

Taking care of yourself

Supporting someone through a long taper is real work. It is not the same work as being the person tapering, but it is not negligible.

Your own sleep, your own routines, your own connections outside the household, and your own occasional breaks are as important during their taper as they are at any other time. Do not deprioritise yourself in an attempt to be the perfect supporter. A stable partner or family member with their own life intact is more useful than an exhausted one who has given up their own routines to worry more.

If you find that the taper is affecting you more than you expected, or that you are struggling with your own mood or sleep, this is worth naming. Talking to a therapist, a trusted friend, or a peer community for supporters can help. The main crisis lines listed in Appendix F are for you too, if you need them.

A short closing note

Your person chose to come off, or is trying to come off, for their own reasons. They may not always be able to articulate those reasons when the process is hard. Trust that they had them. Trust that they are working with their prescriber and doing their best.

What they need from you is not a saviour. What they need is a steady presence, a household that stays reasonably stable, and someone who does not fold when things are difficult. Being that person is a real form of support, and it matters more than any single intervention.

Thank you for being with them through this.

References

Chouinard, G., & Chouinard, V.-A. (2015). New classification of selective serotonin reuptake inhibitor withdrawal. Psychotherapy and Psychosomatics, 84(2), 63 to 71.

Davies, J., & Read, J. (2019). A systematic review into the incidence, severity and duration of antidepressant withdrawal effects: Are guidelines evidence-based? Addictive Behaviors, 97, 111 to 121.

Fava, G. A. (2020). May antidepressant drugs worsen the conditions they are supposed to treat? The clinical foundations of the oppositional model of tolerance. Therapeutic Advances in Psychopharmacology, 10.

Fava, G. A., & Belaise, C. (2018). Discontinuing antidepressant drugs: Lesson from a failed trial and extensive clinical experience. Psychotherapy and Psychosomatics, 87(5), 257 to 267.

Fava, G. A., Gatti, A., Belaise, C., Guidi, J., & Offidani, E. (2015). Withdrawal symptoms after selective serotonin reuptake inhibitor discontinuation: A systematic review. Psychotherapy and Psychosomatics, 84(2), 72 to 81.

Fava, G. A., Guidi, J., Rafanelli, C., & Sonino, N. (2015). The clinical inadequacy of evidence-based medicine and the need for a conceptual framework based on clinical judgment. Psychotherapy and Psychosomatics, 84(1), 1 to 3.

Framer, A. (2021). What I have learnt from helping thousands of people taper off antidepressants and other psychotropic medications. Therapeutic Advances in Psychopharmacology, 11.

Groot, P. C., & van Os, J. (2020). How user knowledge of psychotropic drug withdrawal resulted in the development of person-specific tapering medication. Therapeutic Advances in Psychopharmacology, 10.

Guy, A., Brown, M., Lewis, S., & Horowitz, M. (2020). The 'patient voice': Patients who experience antidepressant withdrawal symptoms are often dismissed, or misdiagnosed with relapse, or a new medical condition. Therapeutic Advances in Psychopharmacology, 10.

Hengartner, M. P., Schulthess, L., Sorensen, A., & Framer, A. (2020). Protracted withdrawal syndrome after stopping antidepressants: A descriptive quantitative analysis of consumer narratives from a large internet forum. Therapeutic Advances in Psychopharmacology, 10.

Horowitz, M. A., & Taylor, D. (2019). Tapering of SSRI treatment to mitigate withdrawal symptoms. The Lancet Psychiatry, 6(6), 538 to 546.

Horowitz, M. A., & Taylor, D. (2022). Distinguishing relapse from antidepressant withdrawal: Clinical pràctice and antidepressant discontinuation studies. BJPsych Advances, 28(5), 297 to 311. https://doi.org/10.1192/bja.2021.62

Horowitz, M. A., & Taylor, D. (2024). Deprescribing guidelines for antidepressants, benzodiazepines, gabapentinoids and z-drugs. Wiley-Blackwell.

Horowitz, M. A., Framer, A., Hengartner, M. P., Sorensen, A., & Taylor, D. (2023). Estimating risk of antidepressant withdrawal from a review of published data. CNS Drugs, 37(2), 143 to 157.

Mahmood, R., Wallace, V., Wiles, N., Kessler, D., Button, K. S., & Fairchild, G. (2024). The lived experience of withdrawal from selective serotonin reuptake inhibitor (SSRI) antidepressants: A qualitative interview study. Health

Expectations, 27(1), e13966. https://doi.org/10.1111/hex.13966

Moncrieff, J. (2008). The myth of the chemical cure: A critique of psychiatric drug treatment. Palgrave Macmillan.

Read, J., Renton, J., Harrop, C., Geekie, J., & Dowrick, C. (2020). A survey of UK general practitioners about depression, antidepressants and withdrawal: Implementing the 2019 Public Health England report. Therapeutic Advances in Psychopharmacology, 10.

Rennwald, A., & Hengartner, M. P. (2025). Post-acute withdrawal syndrome (PAWS) after stopping antidepressants: A systematic review with meta-narrative synthesis. Epidemiology and Psychiatric Sciences, 34, e29. https://doi.org/10.1017/S204579602500023X

Royal College of Psychiatrists. (2020). Stopping antidepressants (patient information resource).

Ruhe, H. G., Horikx, A., van Avendonk, M., Groeneweg, B. F., & Woutersen-Koch, H. (2019). Tapering of SSRI treatment to mitigate withdrawal symptoms. The Lancet Psychiatry, 6(7), 561 to 562.

Sorensen, A. (2024). Crossing zero: Withdrawing from psychiatric drugs safely. Self-published.

Therapeutics Initiative. (2025, June). Letter 156: Antidepressant withdrawal syndrome, an update. University of British Columbia.

Therapeutics Initiative. (2025, July). Letter 157: How to stop antidepressants. University of British Columbia.

Warner, C. H., Bobo, W., Warner, C., Reid, S., & Rachal, J. (2006). Antidepressant discontinuation syndrome. American Family Physician, 74(3), 449 to 456.

World Health Organization. (2023). Guidance on mental health, human rights and legislation.

www.ingramcontent.com/pod-product-compliance
Lightning Source LLC
LaVergne TN
LVHW022040200926
848481LV00003B/723
9798905991936